THE
CELLULAR
HEALTH
COOKBOOK

Scientifically Proven Recipes Inspired by the
Knowledge of Dr. Mercola, for Longevity,
Overall Well-Being and Joy

By
Elisa M. Timm

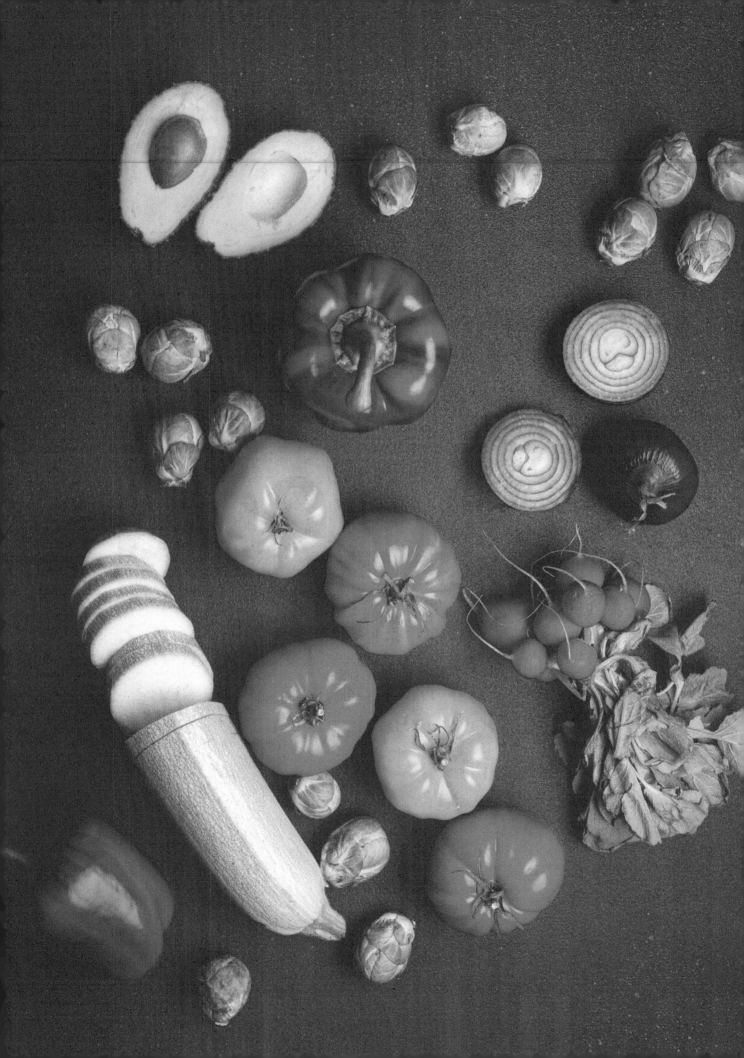

COPYRIGHT PAGE

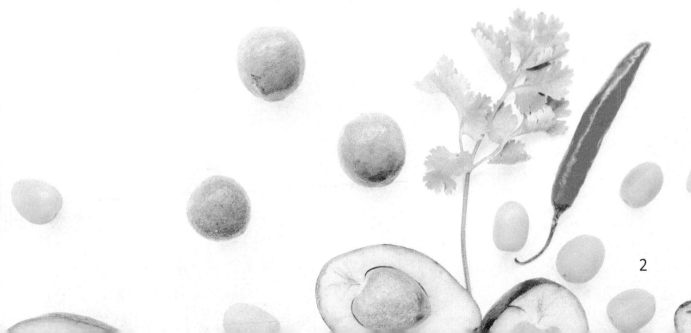

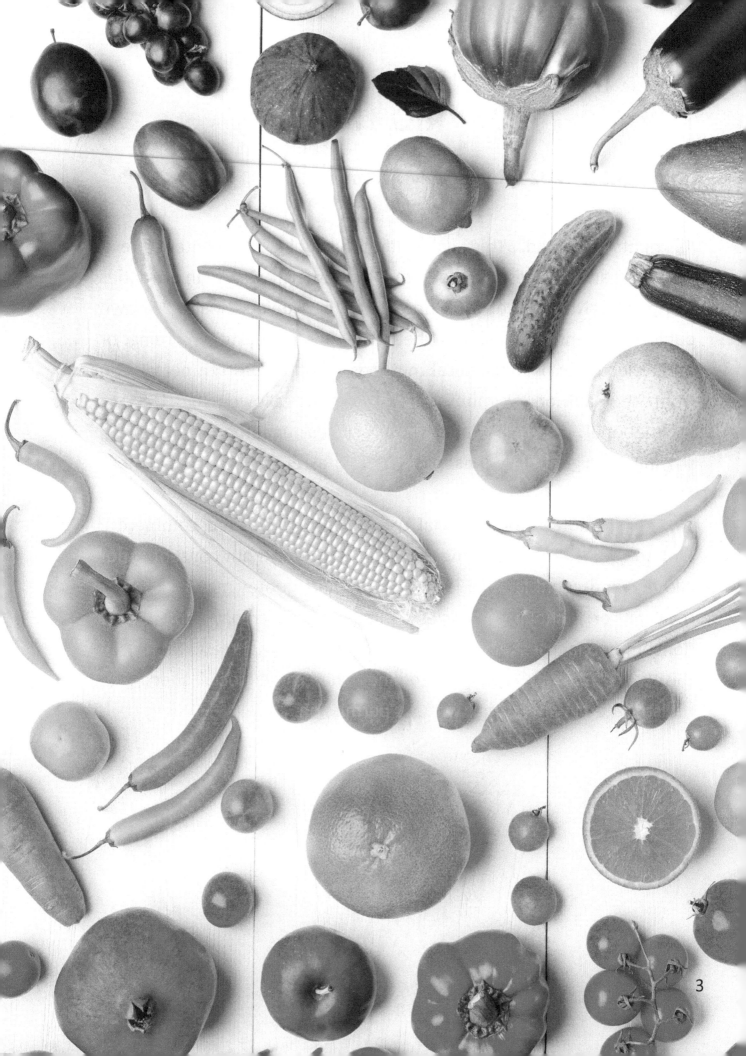

TABLE OF CONTENTS

INTRODUCTION

Our bodies are composed of trillions of cells, each playing a critical role in maintaining our overall health, energy levels, and vitality. Cells are the basic building blocks of life—responsible for generating energy, repairing damage, and supporting every . function within our bodies. At the core of health and longevity lies cellular health. When our cells function optimally, they contribute to a strong immune system, enhanced metabolism, and even longevity. Conversely, when cellular health is compromised, it can lead to chronic diseases, accelerated aging, and fatigue.

The modern lifestyle, characterized by processed foods, stress, environmental toxins, and a lack of physical activity, often leads to cellular damage. This damage primarily occurs due to inflammation, oxidative stress (caused by free radicals), and poor nutrition. Therefore, the key to slowing down aging and preventing disease is ensuring that our cells are nourished, protected, and capable of regenerating efficiently.

HOW NUTRITION IMPACTS CELLULAR LONGEVITY

Food is not just fuel; it is information that our cells use to function. Every bite we take influences cellular processes. For example, certain nutrients support mitochondrial function—the powerhouse of our cells—while others play roles in reducing oxidative stress, promoting DNA repair, or fighting inflammation. The right nutrition can directly influence how well our cells function and how resilient they are against damage.

Here are some ways nutrition impacts cellular health:

- **Antioxidants Combat Oxidative Stress**

Oxidative stress occurs when there is an imbalance between free radicals and antioxidants in the body. Free radicals are unstable molecules that can damage cells, leading to aging and various diseases. Antioxidants, found in fruits, vegetables, and certain superfoods, neutralize these free radicals, protecting cells from damage. Ingredients like berries, leafy greens, and nuts are rich in antioxidants such as vitamin C, vitamin E, and polyphenols, which protect the integrity of cellular structures.

- **Healthy Fats Support Cell Membrane Integrity**

Every cell in our body is surrounded by a membrane made up of fat molecules. The quality of fats we consume directly affects the flexibility and function of these membranes. Omega-3 fatty acids, found in foods like salmon, flaxseeds, and walnuts, help maintain the fluidity and health of cell membranes, allowing for optimal communication between cells and efficient nutrient transport.

- **Protein for Cellular Repair and Regeneration**

Protein provides the essential building blocks, known as amino acids, that are necessary for the repair and regeneration of cells. High-quality proteins from sources like lean meats, fish, beans, and legumes are crucial for the synthesis of enzymes, hormones, and tissues. Collagen-rich foods also support the regeneration of skin cells, tendons, and cartilage.

- **Phytochemicals and Cellular Defense**

Phytochemicals are naturally occurring compounds found in plants that have protective effects on cells. Compounds like flavonoids, carotenoids, and polyphenols have been shown to enhance cellular defense mechanisms, reduce inflammation, and even promote autophagy—a process where cells break down and remove damaged components, allowing for cellular renewal.

- **Fiber and Cellular Detoxification**

A diet rich in fiber supports healthy digestion, which in turn aids in the detoxification of harmful substances that can damage cells. Soluble and insoluble fibers found in fruits, vegetables, and whole grains help bind to toxins and waste products, promoting their removal from the body and reducing the risk of cellular inflammation.

A GUIDE TO USING THIS COOKBOOK

This cookbook is more than just a collection of recipes; it is a comprehensive guide to nourishing your cells from the inside out. The recipes within are designed to be both delicious and functional, using ingredients that specifically target and enhance cellular health. From antioxidant-rich meals to protein-packed dishes for cellular repair, each recipe serves a purpose in maintaining cellular vitality.

Here's how to get the most out of **"The Cellular Health Cookbook"**:

- **Ingredient Spotlight:** At the beginning of each chapter, you'll find a list of key ingredients used in the recipes, along with their specific benefits for cellular health. This will help you understand why certain foods are included and how they contribute to your overall well-being.
- **Practical Meal Planning:** The book is organized to provide a balance of breakfast, lunch, dinner, and snack options that fit easily into your daily life. Each recipe is designed to maximize nutrient absorption while promoting energy, repair, and longevity.
- **Flexible Recipes:** Many recipes are adaptable to various dietary preferences, including plant-based, low-carb, and anti-inflammatory options. Whether you're seeking to boost energy, reduce inflammation, or support detoxification, there are flexible choices to suit your needs.
- **Meal Plans for Longevity:** In addition to individual recipes, this cookbook provides meal plans for specific health goals, such as reducing inflammation, improving gut health, and boosting energy levels.

KEY INGREDIENTS FOR CELLULAR HEALTH

To build and maintain healthy cells, your body needs a variety of essential nutrients. The following are some of the key ingredients you'll encounter in this cookbook, along with their benefits for cellular health:

Berries (Blueberries, Raspberries, Acai)

- Rich in antioxidants, particularly anthocyanins, which help protect cells from oxidative stress. They are also anti-inflammatory and promote healthy brain function.

Leafy Greens (Kale, Spinach, Swiss Chard)

- Packed with vitamins A, C, and K, as well as minerals like magnesium and potassium, which are critical for cellular energy production and detoxification.

Cruciferous Vegetables (Broccoli, Cauliflower, Brussels Sprouts)

- High in sulforaphane, a compound that supports the body's detoxification processes and boosts cellular defense mechanisms.

Healthy Fats (Avocado, Olive Oil, Nuts)

- Provide omega-3 fatty acids, which enhance the fluidity of cell membranes, support brain health, and reduce inflammation.

Probiotic Foods (Yogurt, Kefir, Sauerkraut)

- Contain beneficial bacteria that support gut health, which in turn enhances nutrient absorption and strengthens the immune system.

Wild-Caught Fish (Salmon, Sardines, Mackerel)

- Rich in omega-3 fatty acids, these fish support heart health, reduce inflammation, and promote brain function.

Spices and Herbs (Turmeric, Ginger, Garlic)

- Potent anti-inflammatory and antioxidant properties that protect cells from damage and support overall cellular regeneration.

Nuts and Seeds (Walnuts, Chia Seeds, Flaxseeds)

- Provide essential fatty acids and antioxidants that promote brain health, heart health, and cellular repair.

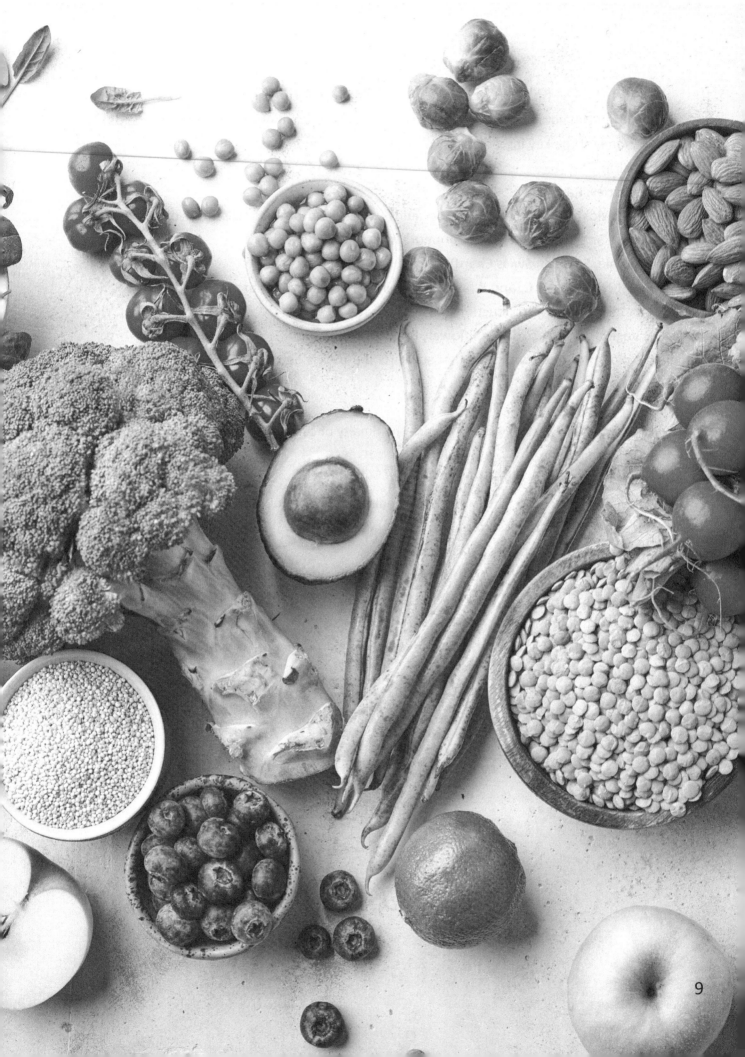

THE FOUNDATIONS OF CELLULAR NUTRITION

Achieving and maintaining optimal cellular health requires an understanding of the building blocks that support every function in our bodies. This chapter explores three critical pillars of cellular nutrition: macronutrients and micronutrients, superfoods for cellular repair, and the importance of hydration and detoxification. By the end, you'll have a solid foundation in how to nourish your cells for peak health, longevity, and vitality.

UNDERSTANDING MACRONUTRIENTS AND MICRONUTRIENTS

Macronutrients—proteins, fats, and carbohydrates—are the primary sources of energy for our bodies and provide the structural components needed for cellular repair and growth. Micronutrients, on the other hand, include vitamins, minerals, and trace elements that support various biochemical processes essential for cellular function.

1. Macronutrients: The Building Blocks of Cellular Health

- **Proteins**: The Body's Repair and Regeneration Agents Proteins are the most important macronutrient when it comes to cellular repair and growth. Made up of amino acids, proteins are responsible for creating the enzymes that power cellular reactions, building tissues like muscles and skin, and supporting the immune system.

Key Functions of Proteins for Cellular Health:

- Amino Acids: Proteins are broken down into amino acids, which are used to build new proteins that repair damaged cells, produce enzymes, and create structural components such as collagen.
- Enzymatic Reactions: Many enzymes that facilitate vital biochemical reactions in cells are proteins. These enzymes assist in everything from digesting food to repairing DNA.
- Immune Support: Protein is essential for producing antibodies and white blood cells, which are critical for defending the body against pathogens and repairing cellular damage caused by infections.

Sources of Cellular Health-Boosting Proteins:

- Lean Meats: Chicken, turkey, and lean beef provide complete proteins with all essential amino acids.
- Fish: Wild-caught salmon and sardines are rich in protein and omega-3 fatty acids that reduce inflammation.
- Legumes: Beans, lentils, and chickpeas are excellent plant-based protein sources that provide fiber and other essential nutrients.

- **Fats**: Supporting Cell Membranes and Energy Storage While fats are often misunderstood, they are vital to cellular health. Fats, especially the essential fatty acids, are critical for the integrity of cell membranes, hormone production, and energy storage.

Key Functions of Fats for Cellular Health:

- Cell Membrane Structure: Every cell is surrounded by a membrane composed of lipids (fats). Healthy fats like omega-3s (found in fish and flaxseeds) make cell membranes more flexible and efficient at regulating the passage of nutrients and waste.
- Hormone Production: Fats are essential for producing hormones, including those that regulate metabolism and inflammation, such as cortisol and testosterone.
- Inflammation Regulation: Omega-3 fatty acids reduce chronic inflammation, which can damage cells and accelerate aging. These healthy fats also support brain cell function, helping to prevent cognitive decline.

Sources of Cellular Health-Boosting Fats:

- Avocados: A rich source of monounsaturated fats that support healthy cell membranes.
- Nuts and Seeds: Walnuts, flaxseeds, and chia seeds provide omega-3 fatty acids and other nutrients essential for reducing inflammation and maintaining heart health.
- Olive Oil: Extra virgin olive oil contains high levels of monounsaturated fats and antioxidants that protect cells from oxidative stress.

- **Carbohydrates**: Fueling Cellular Energy Carbohydrates are the body's primary source of energy. Once digested, carbohydrates are converted into glucose, which fuels cellular activities. However, the type of carbohydrates you consume matters.

Key Functions of Carbohydrates for Cellular Health:

- Energy Production: Cells, particularly in the brain and muscles, rely on glucose for quick energy. Complex carbohydrates, like whole grains and vegetables, release glucose slowly, providing sustained energy throughout the day.
- Fiber for Cellular Detoxification: Although fiber is a carbohydrate, it is indigestible. It plays a crucial role in supporting digestive health by aiding in the removal of toxins, preventing cellular damage caused by harmful waste products.

Sources of Cellular Health-Boosting Carbohydrates:

- Whole Grains: Brown rice, quinoa, and oats provide complex carbohydrates and fiber, which support steady energy levels and promote healthy digestion.
- Vegetables: Leafy greens, root vegetables, and cruciferous vegetables offer carbohydrates along with a high concentration of vitamins, minerals, and antioxidants.
- Fruits: Berries, apples, and citrus fruits are rich in fiber, vitamins, and natural sugars that provide cellular energy without causing spikes in blood sugar levels.

2. Micronutrients: The Essential Nutrients for Cellular Function

While macronutrients supply the body with energy and building blocks, micronutrients—vitamins and minerals—are equally important. These nutrients drive many of the body's most critical processes, including immune function, DNA repair, and energy production.

- **Vitamins: The Catalysts for Cellular Processes**
  - Vitamin C: This powerful antioxidant protects cells from oxidative damage caused by free radicals. It is also essential for collagen synthesis, which supports skin, tendons, and other connective tissues. Sources include citrus fruits, berries, and bell peppers.
  - Vitamin D: Critical for calcium absorption and immune function, vitamin D also supports the health of cell membranes and aids in cellular differentiation. It is found in fatty fish and can be synthesized by the body through sunlight exposure.
  - B-Vitamins: B-vitamins, such as B12, B6, and folate, are involved in energy production at the cellular level. They help convert food into usable energy and are essential for brain function and DNA repair. Sources include leafy greens, eggs, and legumes.
  - Vitamin E: Another potent antioxidant, vitamin E helps protect cell membranes from damage and supports skin and eye health. It is found in nuts, seeds, and leafy greens.

- **Minerals: Building Blocks and Regulators**
  - Magnesium: This mineral plays a role in over 300 enzymatic reactions, including those involved in energy production, muscle function, and nerve signaling. It also supports DNA repair. Good sources of magnesium include dark leafy greens, nuts, and seeds.
  - Zinc: Essential for immune function and DNA synthesis, zinc is critical for cellular repair and regeneration. It is found in shellfish, beef, and pumpkin seeds.
  - Calcium: Not only is calcium essential for bone health, but it also plays a role in muscle function and cellular communication. Dairy products, leafy greens, and fortified plant-based milks are excellent sources of calcium.
  - Iron: Iron is necessary for the production of hemoglobin, which carries oxygen to cells. Without enough iron, cells cannot function properly, leading to fatigue and impaired cellular energy production. Good sources of iron include red meat, lentils, and spinach.

SUPERFOODS FOR CELLULAR REPAIR

Superfoods are nutrient-dense foods that provide a wealth of vitamins, minerals, antioxidants, and other compounds that support cellular health. Incorporating these superfoods into your diet can boost cellular repair, reduce inflammation, and protect against oxidative damage.

- **Berries: Antioxidant Powerhouses**
  - Blueberries: Rich in anthocyanins and vitamin C, blueberries protect cells from oxidative stress, support brain health, and may even promote the repair of DNA damage caused by free radicals.

- Goji Berries: Known for their high levels of antioxidants, goji berries also contain essential amino acids and polysaccharides that support immune function and protect cells from damage.
- **Leafy Greens: Cellular Detoxification and Vitality**
  - Kale: High in vitamins A, C, and K, kale is a powerful anti-inflammatory food that helps detoxify cells and supports overall health.
  - Spinach: Packed with iron, magnesium, and vitamins, spinach helps boost energy levels, supports cellular repair, and protects against oxidative damage.
- **Cruciferous Vegetables: Detoxifiers and Protectors**
  - Broccoli: Rich in sulforaphane, a compound that enhances the body's detoxification enzymes, broccoli helps remove toxins and supports cellular defense mechanisms.
  - Brussels Sprouts: Another cruciferous vegetable high in antioxidants and fiber, Brussels sprouts promote healthy digestion and protect cells from oxidative damage.
- **Nuts and Seeds: Healthy Fats and Antioxidants**
  - Almonds: A great source of vitamin E, almonds help protect cell membranes from oxidative damage and promote skin health.
  - Chia Seeds: Packed with omega-3 fatty acids, fiber, and antioxidants, chia seeds support brain function, reduce inflammation, and promote heart health.
- **Turmeric: Anti-Inflammatory Power**
  - Curcumin, the active compound in turmeric, has been shown to reduce inflammation at the cellular level, protect cells from oxidative damage, and support immune function.

HYDRATION AND DETOXIFICATION FOR CELLULAR HEALTH

Proper hydration is essential for maintaining cellular function and supporting detoxification processes. Water serves as a medium for cellular chemical reactions, helps transport nutrients, and facilitates the removal of waste products.

- **Water: The Foundation of Cellular Health**
  - Cells require water to perform biochemical reactions, generate energy, and remove waste. Dehydration impairs these functions, leading to cellular stress and damage. Drinking adequate amounts of water ensures that your cells remain

MEAL PLANS FOR CELLULAR HEALTH

Incorporating meals that support cellular health is not just about what you eat, but how consistently you nourish your body with the right nutrients. This chapter provides three carefully curated meal plans aimed at supporting specific aspects of cellular health: reducing inflammation, detoxifying the body, and giving your cells a quick nutrient boost. These plans ensure that you not only meet your daily nutritional needs but also target underlying cellular processes essential for vitality and longevity.

Each meal plan focuses on delivering the right balance of macronutrients (proteins, healthy fats, and complex carbohydrates) and micronutrients (vitamins, minerals, and phytochemicals) to optimize cellular function. Whether you're dealing with inflammation, looking to detox, or seeking a quick health boost, these plans offer practical, easy-to-follow solutions.

7-Day Anti-Inflammatory Meal Plan

Chronic inflammation is one of the leading causes of cellular damage. It can contribute to a host of health issues, from cardiovascular disease to autoimmune disorders. The goal of this anti-inflammatory meal plan is to minimize inflammatory triggers while boosting your intake of foods that combat inflammation at the cellular level.

This plan emphasizes foods rich in antioxidants, omega-3 fatty acids, and anti-inflammatory compounds such as polyphenols and flavonoids. Key ingredients include fatty fish, berries, leafy greens, nuts, seeds, and turmeric. Avoidance of processed foods, sugars, and refined carbohydrates is essential to allow your cells to repair and rejuvenate.

Day 1:

Breakfast:

- Chia Seed Pudding with Blueberries and Almond Butter
  - Rich in omega-3s and antioxidants, this breakfast reduces inflammation and supports brain function.

Lunch:

- Spinach Salad with Grilled Salmon, Avocado, and Walnuts
  - Salmon and walnuts provide anti-inflammatory omega-3s, while avocado offers healthy fats to support cell membranes.

Snack:

- Sliced Apples with Turmeric-Spiced Hummus
  - The curcumin in turmeric is a powerful anti-inflammatory compound, and apples add fiber for gut health.

Dinner:

- Lemon-Roasted Chicken with Quinoa and Steamed Broccoli
  - Lean protein from the chicken supports cell repair, while broccoli contains sulforaphane, a compound known to enhance cellular detoxification.

Hydration:

- Herbal Tea with Ginger and Lemon
  - Ginger is known for its anti-inflammatory properties and can help soothe the digestive system.

Day 2:

Breakfast:

- Green Smoothie with Spinach, Flaxseeds, and Pineapple
  - This fiber-rich smoothie provides antioxidants and supports gut health, which is vital for reducing inflammation.

Lunch:

- Sweet Potato and Black Bean Bowl with Cilantro-Lime Dressing
  - Rich in fiber and antioxidants, sweet potatoes help regulate blood sugar, while black beans provide plant-based protein for cellular repair.

Snack:

- Carrot Sticks with Tahini Dip
  - Carrots offer beta-carotene, an antioxidant that reduces inflammation, while tahini provides healthy fats and minerals.

Dinner:

- Baked Cod with Olive Oil, Garlic, and Wilted Kale
  - Cod is a lean, anti-inflammatory protein, and kale is packed with vitamins A, C, and K, essential for immune function and cellular repair.

Hydration:

- Green Tea with a Squeeze of Lemon
  - Green tea is rich in polyphenols, which help lower inflammation and oxidative stress.

Day 3:

Breakfast:

- Overnight Oats with Chia Seeds, Almond Milk, and Strawberries
  - Strawberries are loaded with vitamin C, which supports collagen production and reduces inflammation.

Lunch:

- Quinoa Salad with Roasted Vegetables and Pumpkin Seeds
  - Quinoa is a complete protein, and roasted vegetables provide fiber and antioxidants that promote cellular health.

Snack:

- Celery Sticks with Guacamole
- Avocados contain healthy fats that support brain health and reduce inflammation, while celery provides hydration and fiber.

Dinner:

- Turmeric-Lentil Soup with Carrots and Spinach
- This soup is a powerhouse of anti-inflammatory ingredients, with turmeric, lentils, and nutrient-dense spinach aiding cellular repair.

Hydration:

- Turmeric-Infused Water
- Drinking turmeric-infused water can help combat inflammation throughout the day.

DETOX AND REGENERATION MEAL PLAN

The body is constantly detoxifying itself through the liver, kidneys, lungs, and skin. However, the accumulation of toxins from environmental factors, processed foods, and stress can hinder these processes and contribute to cellular damage. This meal plan is designed to support the body's natural detoxification pathways while promoting cellular regeneration.

The focus is on whole, unprocessed foods that are high in fiber, antioxidants, and liver-supporting nutrients. Cruciferous vegetables, lemons, beets, and garlic play a central role in this detox and regeneration plan, while avoiding alcohol, caffeine, processed foods, and added sugars is crucial.

Day 1:

Breakfast:

- Warm Lemon Water followed by a Green Smoothie with Kale, Cucumber, and Parsley
  - Lemon water stimulates digestion and detoxifies the liver. Kale and parsley are rich in chlorophyll, helping to cleanse the blood.

Lunch:

- Cabbage and Beet Detox Salad with Apple Cider Vinegar Dressing
  - Cabbage is high in sulfur compounds that support liver detoxification, and beets contain betaine, which aids in liver regeneration.

Snack:

- Raw Carrots with a Sprinkle of Flaxseeds
  - Carrots provide beta-carotene, while flaxseeds support bowel regularity, helping the body to excrete toxins.

Dinner:

- Steamed Broccoli with Garlic and Lemon, Paired with Baked Wild Salmon
  - Broccoli stimulates liver detoxification enzymes, while garlic contains sulfur compounds that enhance cellular regeneration.

Hydration:

- Dandelion Root Tea
  - Dandelion supports liver health and acts as a natural diuretic, helping the body flush out toxins.

Day 2:

Breakfast:

- Smoothie with Spinach, Ginger, Pineapple, and Coconut Water
  - This hydrating, anti-inflammatory smoothie supports digestion and detoxifies the liver.

Lunch:

- Lentil and Kale Soup with Fresh Herbs
  - Lentils are high in fiber and protein, supporting liver and kidney function, while kale aids in detoxification.

Snack:

- Sliced Cucumber and Celery with Olive Tapenade
  - Cucumbers help hydrate and detoxify the body, while olive tapenade provides healthy fats for cellular protection.

Dinner:

- Quinoa-Stuffed Bell Peppers with Roasted Garlic and Basil
  - Quinoa is rich in amino acids, supporting cellular repair, while bell peppers provide vitamin C for detoxification.

Hydration:

- Detox Water with Cucumber, Lemon, and Mint
  - This hydrating drink helps flush out toxins while delivering vitamins that support regeneration.

THE CELLULAR HEALTH PANTRY

The foundation of any healthy diet lies in the ingredients you use, and when it comes to cellular health, certain foods, spices, herbs, and supplements can dramatically enhance your body's ability to repair, regenerate, and function optimally. In this chapter, we'll explore the essential items you should have in your pantry to support your cells. We'll also discuss how to stock your kitchen to ensure you have the necessary components for cellular nutrition, and provide practical tips for sourcing the highest-quality ingredients.

ESSENTIAL SPICES, HERBS, AND SUPPLEMENTS

Spices, herbs, and supplements are much more than flavor enhancers; they offer potent medicinal properties that can protect and restore your cells. These ingredients contain antioxidants, anti-inflammatory compounds, and phytochemicals that help fight oxidative stress, regulate inflammation, and promote detoxification. Below are key spices, herbs, and supplements you should incorporate into your pantry for optimal cellular health.

SPICES FOR CELLULAR HEALTH

- **Turmeric (Curcuma longa)**

Perhaps one of the most potent spices for cellular health, turmeric contains curcumin, a powerful anti-inflammatory compound. Curcumin has been shown to reduce oxidative stress and inflammation at the cellular level, making it essential for preventing cell damage and chronic diseases. Turmeric also promotes autophagy, a process where cells remove damaged components, thereby improving cellular function and longevity.
    - **How to use:** Add turmeric to soups, curries, stir-fries, and smoothies. For better absorption, combine it with black pepper, which enhances curcumin bioavailability by up to 2000%.

- **Ginger (Zingiber officinale)**

Ginger is a potent antioxidant and anti-inflammatory spice known to promote digestive health, reduce inflammation, and protect cells from damage. Its active compounds, such as gingerol, are particularly beneficial for reducing inflammation in the gut, which plays a vital role in nutrient absorption and overall cellular function.
    - **How to use:** Incorporate ginger into teas, smoothies, marinades, and vegetable dishes. Fresh ginger can also be added to juices for a quick cellular health boost.

- **Cinnamon (Cinnamomum verum)**

Rich in antioxidants, cinnamon helps regulate blood sugar levels and reduce inflammation. It has been shown to support mitochondrial health—the energy powerhouse of cells—and may even improve insulin sensitivity, which is crucial for metabolic health.
    - **How to use:** Sprinkle cinnamon on oatmeal, add it to baked goods, or mix it into smoothies and teas.

- **Cayenne Pepper (Capsicum annuum)**

Cayenne contains capsaicin, which stimulates circulation, improves digestion, and aids in detoxification. Capsaicin is also a potent anti-inflammatory and can help reduce oxidative stress by promoting blood flow and oxygen delivery to cells.

  - **How to use:** Add cayenne pepper to soups, stews, and marinades. Use sparingly for heat, but consistently for its health benefits.

- **Black Pepper (Piper nigrum)**

Black pepper enhances the absorption of many nutrients, including curcumin from turmeric. It also contains piperine, which has antioxidant properties and can help protect against oxidative stress in cells.

  - **How to use:** Use black pepper liberally in cooking to enhance nutrient absorption. It pairs well with almost any savory dish.

- **Cardamom (Elettaria cardamomum)**

Cardamom is a warming spice with anti-inflammatory, antioxidant, and detoxifying properties. It aids in digestion, supports liver function, and promotes overall cellular health by reducing inflammation and supporting detoxification pathways.

  - **How to use:** Add cardamom to teas, baked goods, and curries, or use it in conjunction with other warming spices like cinnamon and ginger.

HERBS FOR CELLULAR HEALTH

- **Oregano (Origanum vulgare)**

Oregano is packed with antioxidants and has powerful antimicrobial properties, making it beneficial for supporting the immune system and reducing inflammation. Its active compounds, carvacrol and thymol, protect cells from oxidative stress and support the body's detoxification processes.

  - **How to use:** Use dried or fresh oregano in salads, sauces, and marinades. Oregano oil is also available as a supplement for more concentrated benefits.

- **Rosemary (Rosmarinus officinalis)**

Rosemary is a herb rich in carnosic acid and rosmarinic acid, both of which are powerful antioxidants that protect cells from free radical damage. Rosemary also supports cognitive function by improving blood circulation to the brain.

  - **How to use:** Add fresh or dried rosemary to roasted vegetables, meats, and soups. It can also be infused into oils for dressings or marinades.

- **Thyme (Thymus vulgaris)**

Thyme is another antioxidant-rich herb that supports immune function and reduces inflammation. It contains thymol, which has antibacterial and antifungal properties, supporting a healthy microbiome —critical for nutrient absorption and cellular health.

  - **How to use:** Use thyme in soups, stews, and roasted vegetables, or steep it in hot water for a simple herbal tea.

- **Basil (Ocimum basilicum)**

Basil contains eugenol, a compound with anti-inflammatory and antioxidant properties. Basil is also known to support cellular detoxification processes by enhancing liver function.

- ○ **How to use:** Use fresh basil in salads, pesto, and pasta dishes. Dried basil can be added to soups and sauces for a flavorful antioxidant boost.

- **Mint (Mentha spp.)**

Mint is a refreshing herb with antioxidant and anti-inflammatory properties. It supports digestive health, which is crucial for optimal cellular function, and contains compounds that help reduce oxidative stress.

- ○ **How to use:** Add fresh mint to salads, smoothies, and teas, or use it as a garnish for desserts.

SUPPLEMENTS FOR CELLULAR HEALTH

- **Omega-3 Fatty Acids (Fish Oil, Algal Oil)**

Omega-3s, particularly EPA and DHA, are critical for maintaining the fluidity and integrity of cell membranes. They reduce inflammation and support brain, heart, and joint health. Omega-3s are also essential for mitochondrial function, helping cells produce energy efficiently.

- ○ **How to use:** Take a high-quality fish oil or algal oil supplement daily. Ensure it is free of heavy metals and contaminants for optimal safety and efficacy.

- **Probiotics**

A healthy gut is essential for cellular health, as it facilitates nutrient absorption and helps regulate immune function. Probiotic supplements can support a healthy microbiome, promoting better digestion and reducing systemic inflammation.

- ○ **How to use:** Choose a probiotic supplement with multiple strains and a high CFU (colony-forming units) count. Fermented foods like yogurt, sauerkraut, and kefir can also be natural sources of probiotics.

- **Vitamin D**

Vitamin D is crucial for cellular health as it regulates calcium absorption, supports immune function, and reduces inflammation. It also plays a key role in gene expression and cellular differentiation.

- ○ **How to use:** Take a vitamin D3 supplement, especially if you live in an area with limited sunlight exposure. Combine with a source of healthy fat for better absorption.

- **Magnesium**

Magnesium is involved in over 300 enzymatic processes, including those related to energy production, DNA repair, and muscle function. A magnesium deficiency can impair cellular energy production and contribute to inflammation.

- ○ **How to use:** Supplement with magnesium glycinate or citrate for optimal absorption, or incorporate magnesium-rich foods like leafy greens, nuts, and seeds into your diet.

- **Curcumin (Turmeric Extract)**

If consuming turmeric in foods isn't enough, a curcumin supplement provides concentrated anti-inflammatory benefits. Curcumin supports cellular health by promoting autophagy and reducing chronic inflammation.

- **How to use:** Look for curcumin supplements that contain piperine (black pepper extract) for enhanced absorption.

STOCKING YOUR KITCHEN FOR CELLULAR NUTRITION

Stocking your kitchen with the right ingredients is key to ensuring you're always prepared to cook meals that nourish your cells. A well-organized kitchen not only saves time but also makes it easier to stick to a cellular health-focused diet.

- **Key Staples to Keep in Your Pantry:**
  - **Whole Grains:** Quinoa, brown rice, and oats are excellent sources of fiber, vitamins, and minerals that support cellular health.
  - **Legumes:** Lentils, chickpeas, and beans are rich in plant-based protein, fiber, and essential nutrients that aid in cell repair and regeneration.
  - **Nuts and Seeds:** Almonds, walnuts, chia seeds, and flaxseeds provide healthy fats and antioxidants that protect cells from damage.
  - **Healthy Oils:** Stock your kitchen with extra virgin olive oil, avocado oil, and coconut oil. These oils are rich in healthy fats that support cell membrane integrity and reduce inflammation.
  - **Herbs and Spices:** Keep a variety of fresh and dried herbs and spices on hand to enhance both the flavor and nutritional value of your meals.
  - **Fermented Foods:** Sauerkraut, kimchi, and miso are great for supporting gut health, which is critical for overall cellular function.
  - **Frozen Fruits and Vegetables:** Having frozen options ensures you always have access to antioxidant-rich produce, even when fresh options are limited.

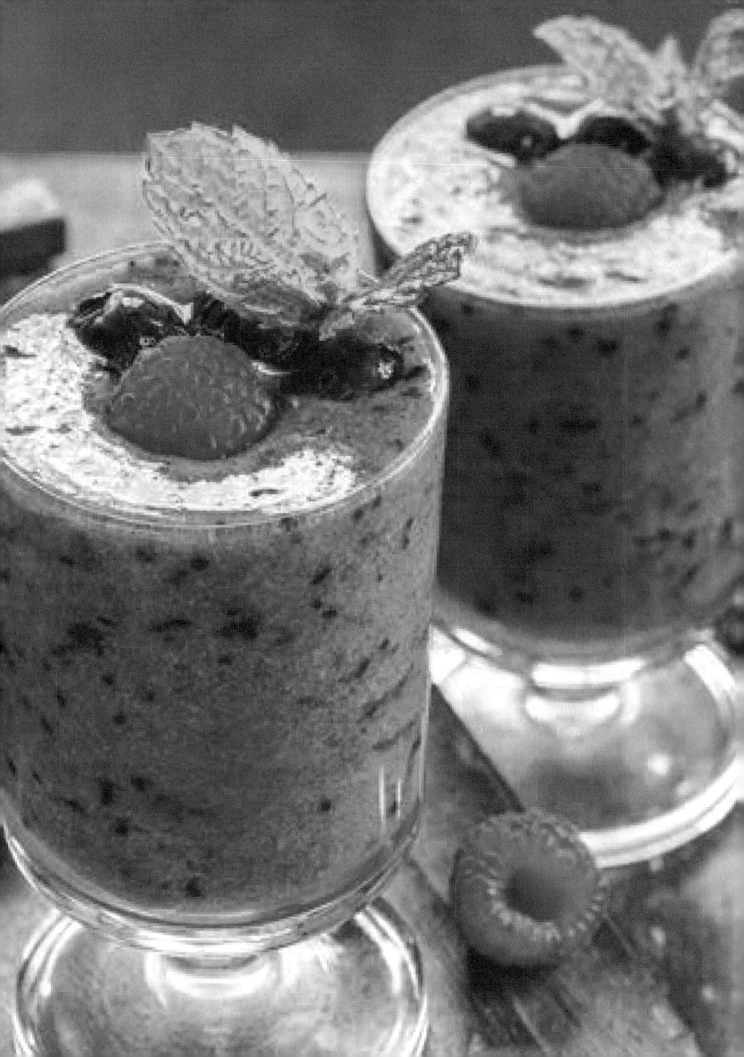

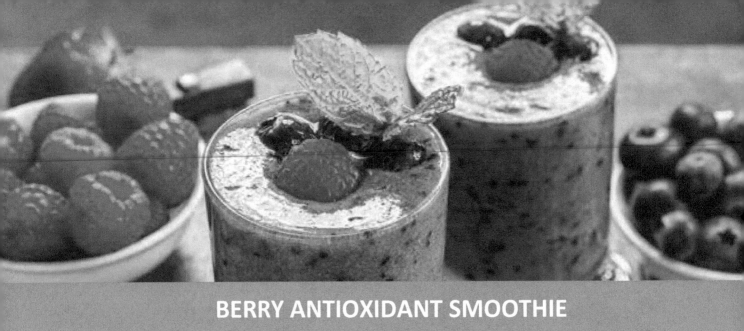

BERRY ANTIOXIDANT SMOOTHIE

Prep Time: 5 Min | **Cook Time: 0 Min** | **Serving Size: 1**

INGREDIENTS:

- 1/2 cup frozen blueberries
- 1/2 cup frozen strawberries
- 1/2 cup frozen raspberries
- 1 small banana
- 1 cup unsweetened almond milk (or any plant-based milk)
- 1 tablespoon chia seeds
- 1/2 teaspoon ground flaxseeds
- 1/4 teaspoon ground cinnamon (optional)
- 1/2 cup spinach (optional, for added nutrients)
- 1 teaspoon honey or maple syrup (optional for sweetness)

INSTRUCTIONS:

- Add the frozen berries, banana, and spinach (if using) to a blender.
- Pour in the almond milk.
- Add chia seeds, ground flaxseeds, and cinnamon (if using).
- Blend on high until smooth and creamy, about 1-2 minutes.
- Taste and adjust sweetness with honey or maple syrup if needed.
- Pour into a glass and enjoy immediately.

NUTRITIONAL FACTS

- Calories: 220
- Total Fat: 6g
- Saturated Fat: 0.5g
- Carbohydrates: 43g
- Fiber: 11g
- Sugars: 21g
- Protein: 5g
- Vitamin C: 90% of the Daily Value (DV)
- Vitamin K: 35% DV
- Calcium: 25% DV
- Iron: 10% DV

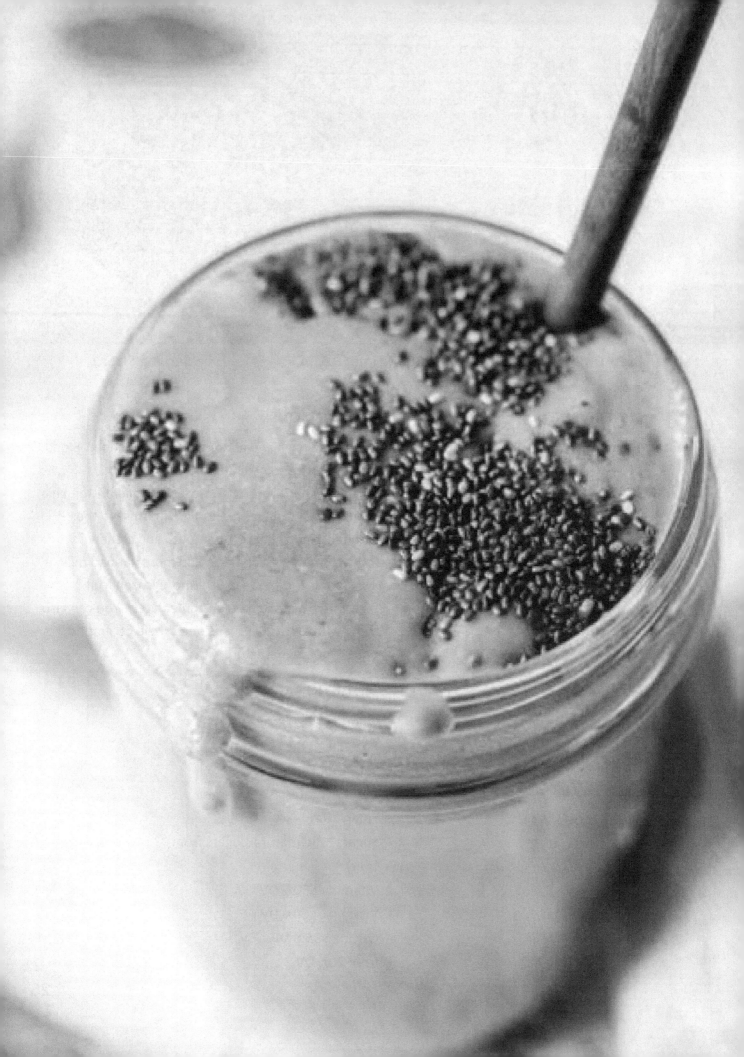

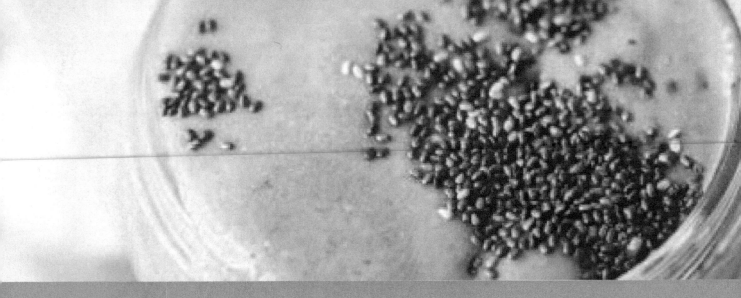

GREEN PROTEIN SMOOTHIE

Prep Time: 5 Min | **Cook Time: 0 Min** | **Serving Size: 1**

INGREDIENTS:

- 1 cup unsweetened almond milk (or any plant-based milk)
- 1 scoop plant-based protein powder (vanilla or unflavored)
- 1 cup spinach (packed)
- ½ banana (frozen for creaminess)
- 1 tablespoon almond butter (or any nut butter)
- 1 tablespoon chia seeds
- ½ cup frozen pineapple or mango chunks
- ½ teaspoon spirulina powder (optional for extra greens)
- Ice cubes (optional for thickness)

INSTRUCTIONS:

- Add the spinach and almond milk to a blender. Blend until smooth and no chunks remain.
- Add the banana, protein powder, almond butter, chia seeds, frozen fruit, and spirulina (if using) to the blender. Blend again until smooth and creamy.
- If the smoothie is too thick, add more almond milk. If it's too thin, add ice cubes or more frozen fruit.
- Pour into a glass and enjoy immediately. You can also top it with extra chia seeds or a drizzle of almond butter for added texture.

NUTRITIONAL FACTS

- Calories: ~320 kcal
- Protein: ~22g
- Fat: ~12g
- Carbohydrates: ~34g
- Fiber: ~9g
- Sugar: ~18g (natural sugars from fruit)
- Vitamin A: 50% DV
- Vitamin C: 60% DV
- Calcium: 35% DV
- Iron: 20% DV

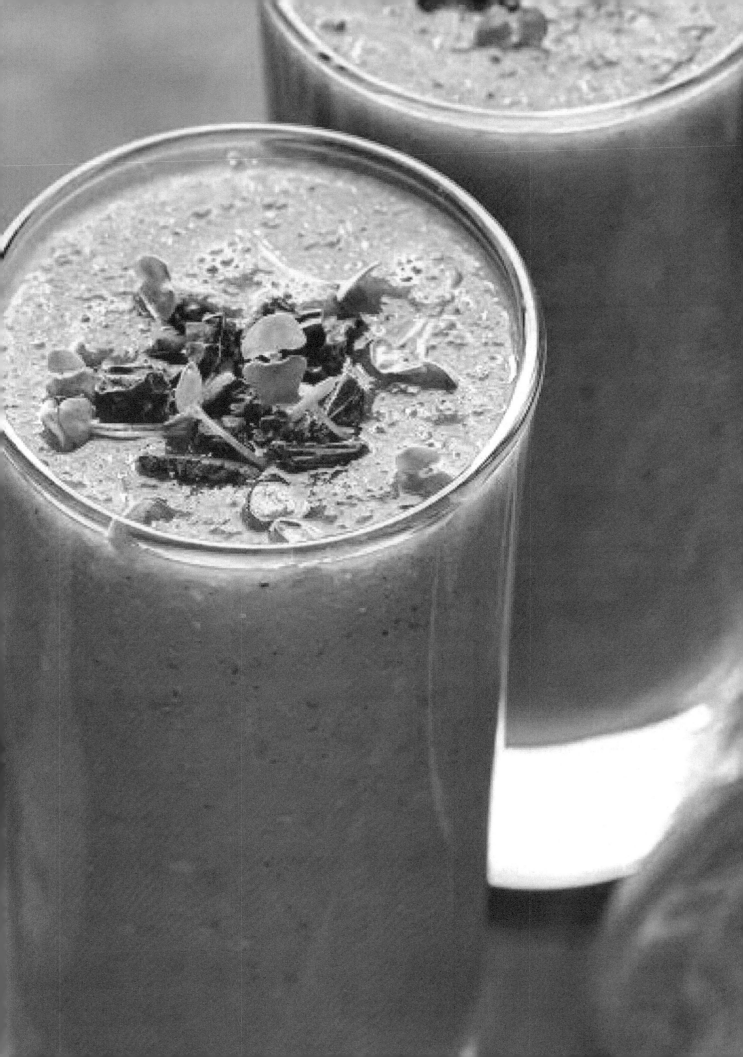

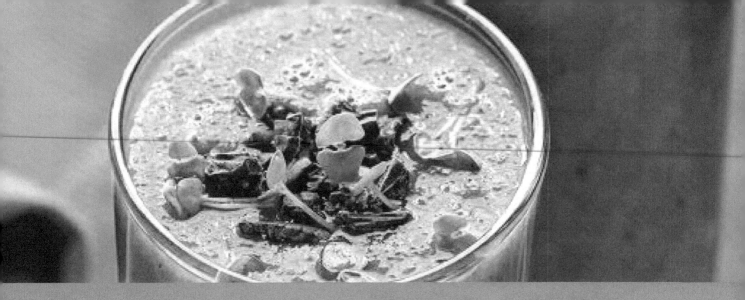

DETOX GREEN JUICE

Prep Time: 10 Min | **Cook Time: 0 Min** | **Serving Size: 2**

INGREDIENTS:

- 2 cups spinach (fresh)
- 1 cucumber (peeled)
- 1 green apple (cored and chopped)
- 1 celery stalk
- 1/2 lemon (peeled)
- 1-inch piece of ginger (peeled)
- 1/2 cup parsley (fresh)
- 1/2 cup water or coconut water (for blending)

NUTRITIONAL FACTS

- Calories: 95
- Protein: 2g
- Carbohydrates: 21g
- Fiber: 6g
- Sugars: 12g
- Fat: 0.5g
- Vitamin C: 65% of Daily Value (DV)
- Vitamin K: 100% of DV
- Potassium: 450mg
- Iron: 15% of DV

INSTRUCTIONS:

- Wash all the vegetables and fruits thoroughly. Peel the cucumber, lemon, and ginger. Core the apple and chop it into smaller pieces.
- Add all the ingredients (spinach, cucumber, green apple, celery, lemon, ginger, parsley, and water) into a blender.
- Start the blender on low, then gradually increase to high speed. Blend until the mixture is smooth.
- If you prefer a smoother juice, pour the blended mixture through a fine mesh strainer or cheesecloth to remove the pulp.
- Pour the juice into a glass and enjoy immediately for maximum freshness and nutritional benefit.

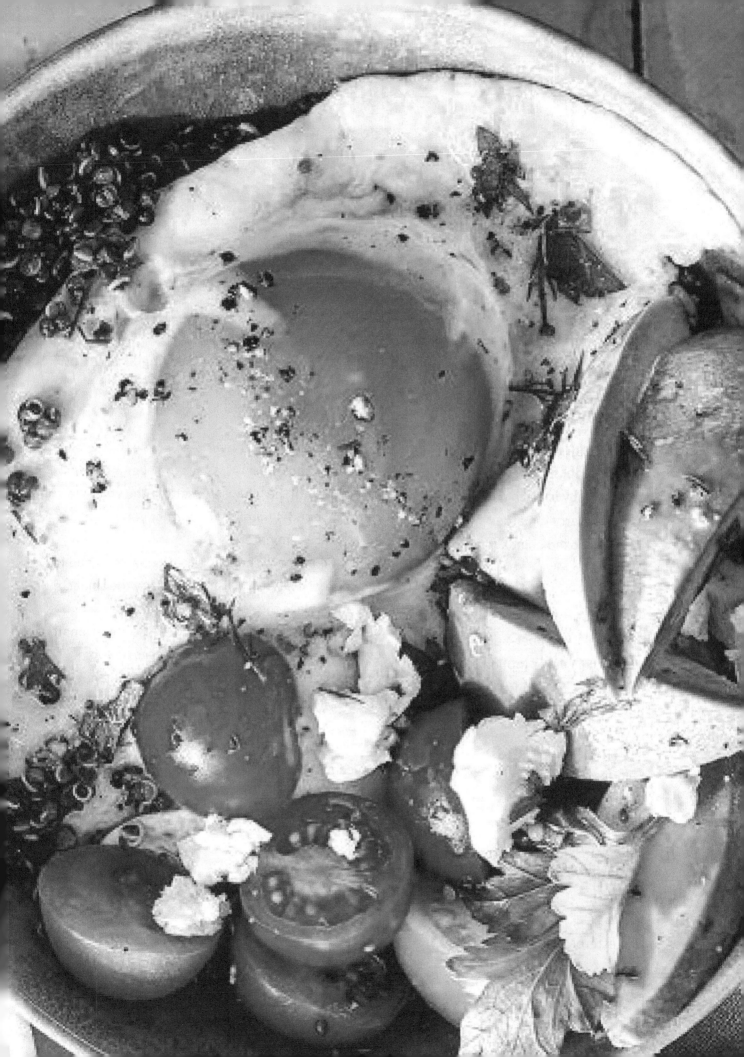

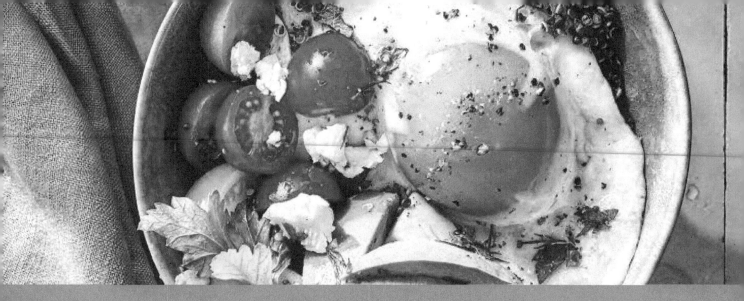

EGG & AVOCADO POWER BOWL

Prep Time: 10 Min | **Cook Time: 10 Min** | **Serving Size: 1 Bowl**

INGREDIENTS:

- 2 large eggs
- 1/2 avocado, sliced
- 1/2 cup baby spinach
- 1/4 cup cherry tomatoes, halved
- 1/4 cup cooked quinoa (optional)
- 1 tbsp olive oil
- 1 tsp lemon juice
- 1/4 tsp sea salt
- 1/4 tsp black pepper
- 1/8 tsp chili flakes (optional)
- Fresh herbs for garnish (optional: parsley, cilantro, or chives)

NUTRITIONAL FACTS

- Calories: 380 kcal
- Protein: 14g
- Fat: 29g (healthy fats from avocado and olive oil)
- Carbohydrates: 18g
- Fiber: 7g
- Sugar: 2g
- Cholesterol: 372mg

INSTRUCTIONS:

- Heat a non-stick skillet over medium heat. Add a bit of olive oil or cooking spray. Crack the eggs into the skillet and cook until the whites are set but the yolks are still runny, about 3-4 minutes. For firmer yolks, cook for an additional 1-2 minutes.
- While the eggs are cooking, slice the avocado and halve the cherry tomatoes. Wash and pat dry the spinach.
- In a bowl, place the cooked quinoa (if using) as the base. Layer the spinach, avocado, and cherry tomatoes over the quinoa. Place the cooked eggs on top.
- Drizzle the olive oil and lemon juice over the bowl. Sprinkle with sea salt, black pepper, and chili flakes (if using).
- Top with fresh herbs for added flavor and visual appeal.
- Serve immediately for a warm, nourishing power bowl.

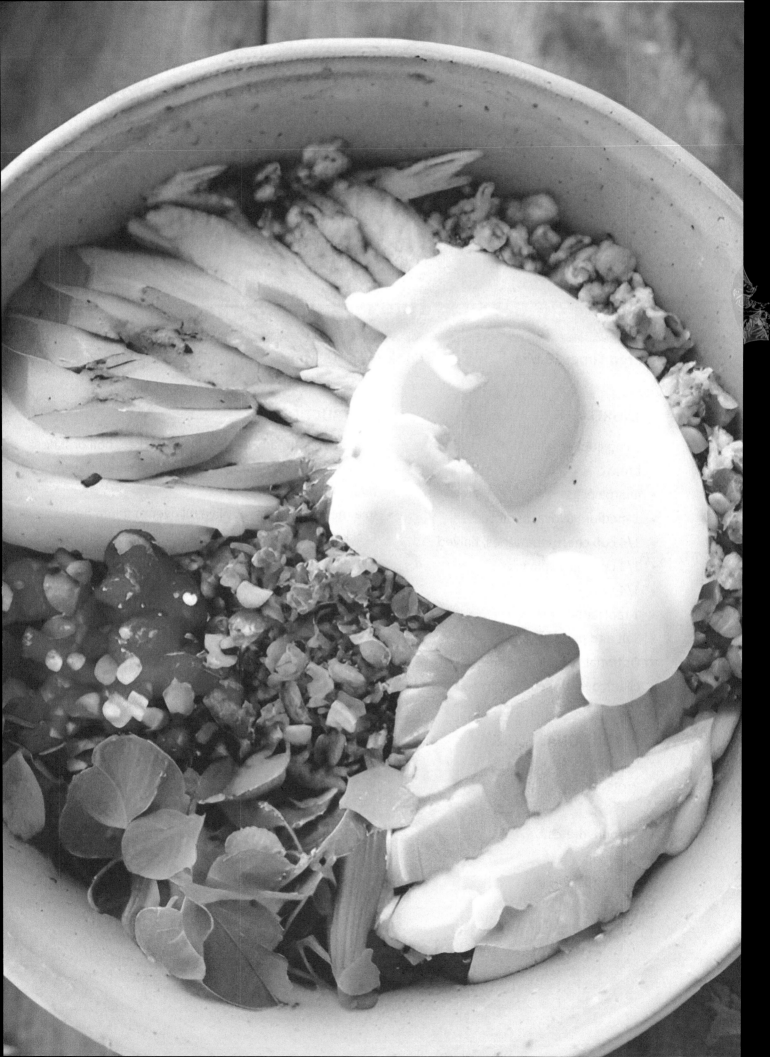

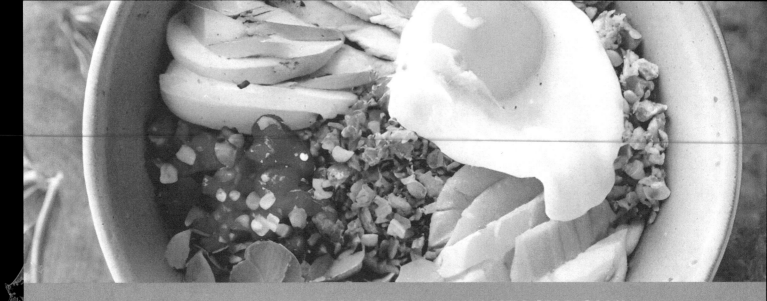

GRAIN-FREE CHICKEN BREAKFAST BOWL

Prep Time: 10 Min | **Cook Time: 15 Min** | **Serving Size: 2**

INGREDIENTS:

- 1 cup cooked, shredded chicken breast
- 4 large eggs
- 1 medium avocado, diced
- 1/4 cup cherry tomatoes, halved
- 1/4 cup baby spinach
- 1/4 teaspoon paprika
- 1 tablespoon olive oil
- Salt and pepper, to taste
- Optional: 1 tablespoon fresh cilantro, chopped

INSTRUCTIONS:

- If you don't already have cooked chicken, boil or bake a chicken breast until fully cooked, then shred it using two forks. Set aside.
- In a medium pan, heat olive oil over medium heat. Crack the eggs into the pan and scramble them until fully cooked. Season with salt, pepper, and paprika.
- In two bowls, divide the scrambled eggs and shredded chicken. Add the diced avocado, cherry tomatoes, and baby spinach.
- Optionally, top with fresh cilantro and an extra sprinkle of salt and pepper to taste. Enjoy immediately.

NUTRITIONAL FACTS

- Calories: 380
- Protein: 30g
- Fat: 27g
- Carbohydrates: 7g
- Fiber: 5g
- Net Carbs: 2g
- Sugars: 1g
- Sodium: 420mg

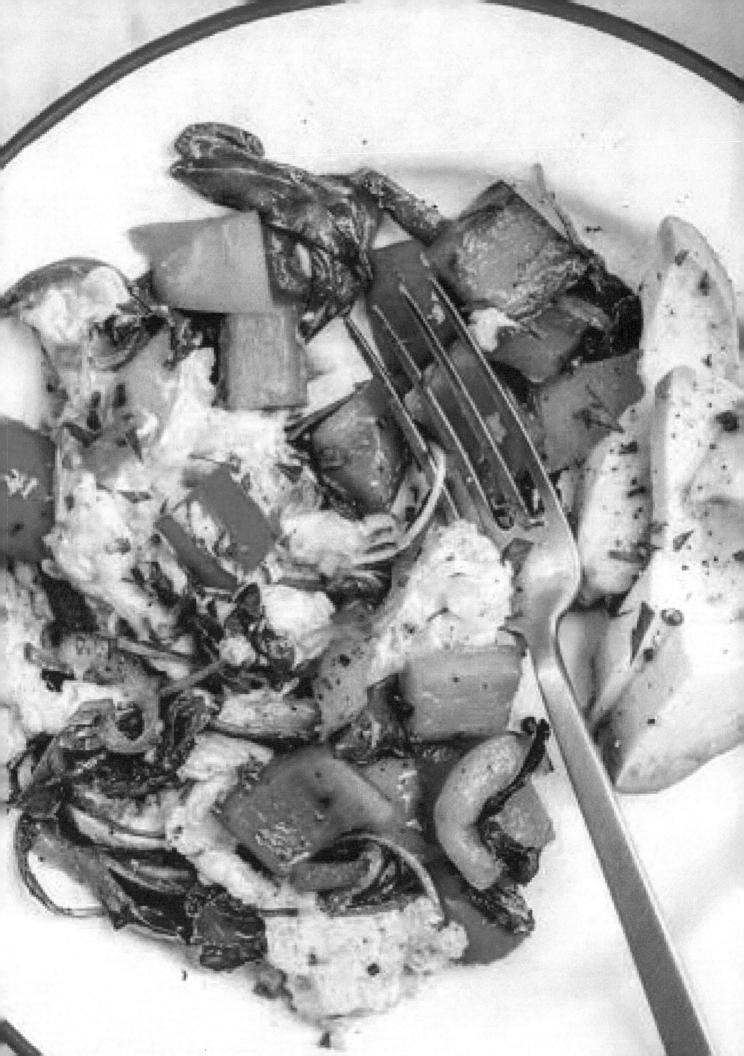

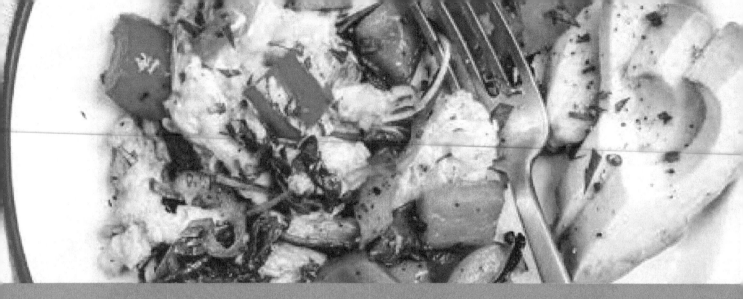

VEGGIE SCRAMBLE

Prep Time: 10 Min | **Cook Time: 10 Min** | **Serving Size: 2**

INGREDIENTS:

- 4 large eggs (or egg substitute for a lighter option)
- 1/4 cup milk (or non-dairy milk)
- 1 cup spinach, chopped
- 1/2 bell pepper, diced (any color)
- 1/2 cup cherry tomatoes, halved
- 1/4 cup onion, diced
- 1/4 cup mushrooms, diced
- 1 tablespoon olive oil or cooking spray
- Salt and pepper, to taste
- Optional toppings: avocado, feta cheese, or fresh herbs (e.g., parsley or cilantro)

NUTRITIONAL FACTS

- Calories: 250kcal
- Protein: 16g
- Fat: 15g
- Carbohydrates: 12g
- Fiber: 3g
- Sugar: 3g

INSTRUCTIONS:

- Chop the spinach, bell pepper, onion, mushrooms, and halve the cherry tomatoes.
- In a mixing bowl, whisk together the eggs and milk. Season with a pinch of salt and pepper.
- Heat olive oil in a non-stick skillet over medium heat. Add the diced onion and bell pepper, and sauté for about 2-3 minutes until they start to soften.
- Stir in the mushrooms, spinach, and cherry tomatoes. Cook for an additional 2-3 minutes until the spinach is wilted and the mushrooms are tender.
- Pour the whisked eggs over the cooked vegetables in the skillet. Let it sit for a few seconds, then gently stir to scramble everything together. Cook for 3-4 minutes or until the eggs are cooked through.
- Remove from heat and serve immediately. Top with optional toppings like avocado, feta cheese, or fresh herbs if desired.

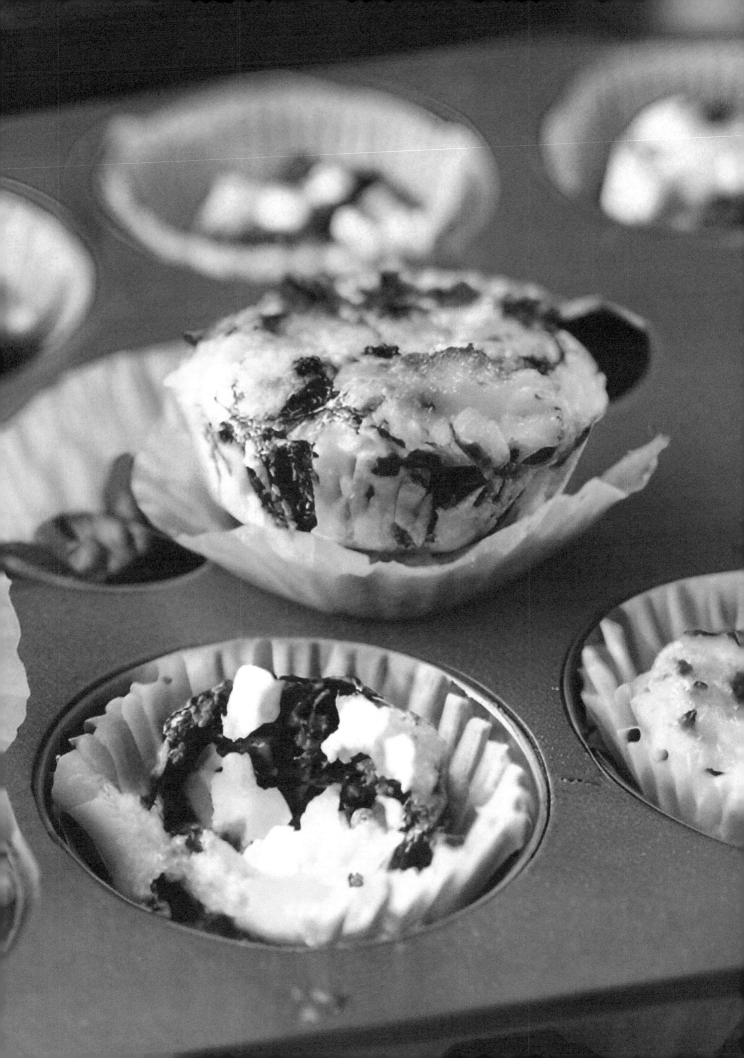

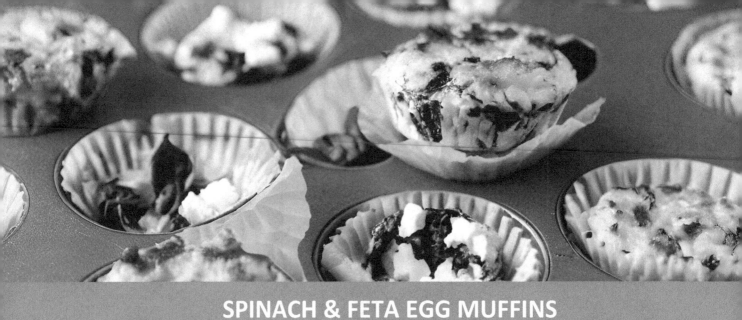

SPINACH & FETA EGG MUFFINS

Prep Time: 10 Min | **Cook Time: 20 Min** | **Serving Size: 12**

INGREDIENTS:

- 6 large eggs
- 1 cup fresh spinach, chopped (or 1/2 cup frozen spinach, thawed and drained)
- 1/2 cup feta cheese, crumbled
- 1/2 cup bell pepper, diced (any color)
- 1/4 cup onion, finely chopped
- 1/4 cup milk (or dairy-free alternative)
- 1/2 teaspoon garlic powder
- 1/2 teaspoon salt
- 1/4 teaspoon black pepper
- Optional: fresh herbs (such as dill or parsley) for garnish

NUTRITIONAL FACTS

- Calories: 100kcal
- Protein: 7g
- Fat: 6g
- Carbohydrates: 4g
- Fiber: 1g
- Sugar: 1g

INSTRUCTIONS:

- Preheat your oven to 350°F (175°C). Grease a muffin tin with cooking spray or line with muffin liners.
- In a large mixing bowl, whisk together the eggs and milk until well combined. Add garlic powder, salt, and black pepper, mixing until incorporated.
- Stir in the chopped spinach, diced bell pepper, onion, and crumbled feta cheese into the egg mixture.
- Pour the egg mixture evenly into the prepared muffin tin, filling each cup about 3/4 full.
- Place the muffin tin in the preheated oven and bake for 18-20 minutes, or until the muffins are set and lightly golden on top.
- Allow the muffins to cool in the pan for a few minutes before carefully removing them. Enjoy warm or store in an airtight container in the fridge for up to a week.

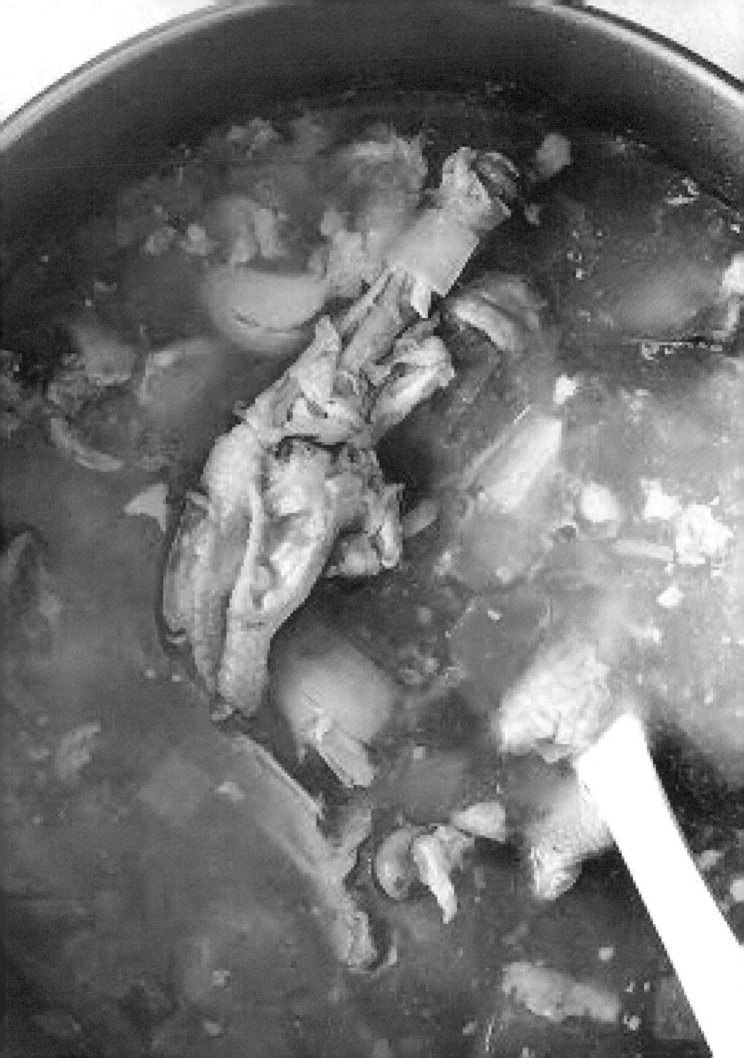

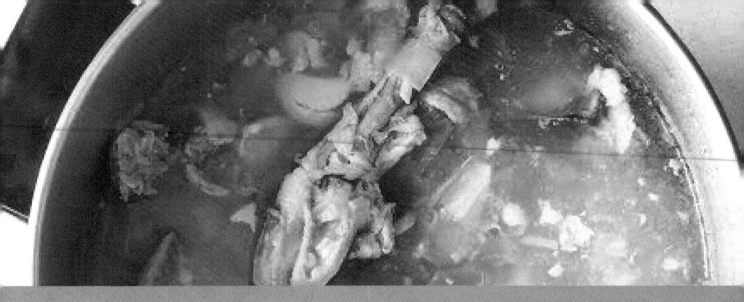

CHICKEN BONE BROTH

Prep Time: 20 Min | **Cook Time: 6 Hours** | **Serving Size: 1 Cup**

INGREDIENTS:

- 2 lbs chicken bones (from a rotisserie chicken or raw bones)
- 2 carrots, chopped
- 2 celery stalks, chopped
- 1 onion, quartered
- 4 cloves garlic, smashed
- 1-2 bay leaves
- 1-2 tablespoons apple cider vinegar (to help extract nutrients from bones)
- Fresh herbs (such as thyme, parsley, or rosemary, optional)
- Salt and pepper to taste
- 10 cups water (or enough to cover the bones)

NUTRITIONAL FACTS

- Calories: 50
- Protein: 8g
- Fat: 2g
- Carbohydrates: 3g
- Fiber: 1g

INSTRUCTIONS:

- If using raw bones, roast them in the oven at 400°F (200°C) for 30 minutes for added flavor.
- Chop the carrots, celery, and onion, and smash the garlic cloves.
- In a slow cooker or a large pot, combine the chicken bones, chopped vegetables, garlic, bay leaves, apple cider vinegar, and any optional herbs.
- Pour in enough water to cover the ingredients (about 10 cups).
- For Slow Cooker: Set it to low and cook for 12-24 hours. The longer it cooks, the more flavorful and nutritious it will be.
- For Stovetop: Bring to a boil, then reduce heat to a simmer. Cover and cook for 4-6 hours. Skim off any foam that rises to the top.
- Once cooked, remove the pot from heat. Strain the broth through a fine-mesh sieve into another pot or large bowl, discarding the solids.
- Let the broth cool before transferring it to jars. You can store it in the refrigerator for up to 5 days or freeze it for longer storage.
- Use the broth as a base for soups, stews, or enjoy it on its own for a warm, nourishing drink.

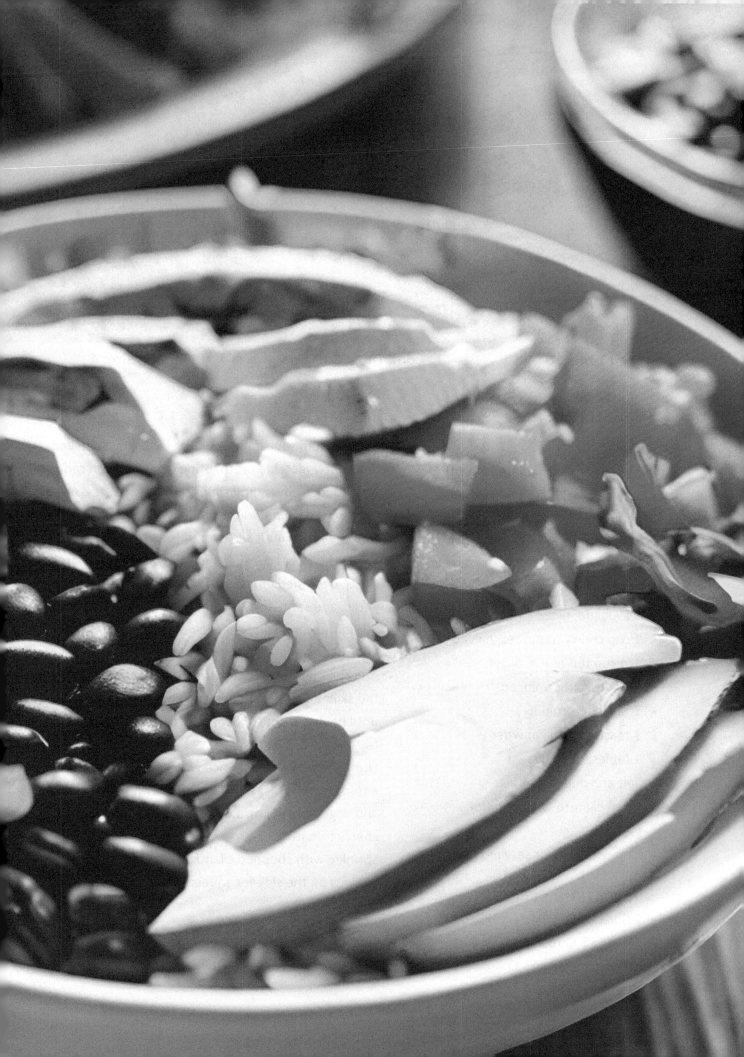

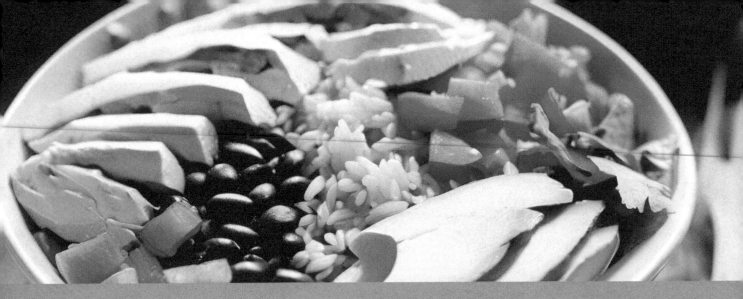

BROWN RICE AND BLACK BEAN BOWL

Prep Time: 10 Min | **Cook Time: 30 Min** | **Serving Size: 4**

INGREDIENTS:

- 1 cup brown rice
- 2 cups water or vegetable broth
- 1 can (15 oz) black beans, drained and rinsed
- 1 cup corn (fresh, frozen, or canned)
- 1 red bell pepper, diced
- 1 avocado, diced
- 1 cup cherry tomatoes, halved
- 1/4 cup red onion, diced
- 2 cloves garlic, minced
- 1 teaspoon cumin
- 1 teaspoon chili powder
- 1 tablespoon olive oil
- Salt and pepper to taste
- Fresh cilantro, chopped (for garnish)
- Lime wedges (for serving)

NUTRITIONAL FACTS

- Calories: 400 | Protein: 15g
- Fat: 15g | Carbohydrates: 60g
- Fiber: 15g | Sugar: 3g

INSTRUCTIONS:

- In a medium saucepan, combine the brown rice and water or vegetable broth. Bring to a boil, then reduce heat to low, cover, and simmer for 30 minutes, or until the rice is tender and the liquid is absorbed. Remove from heat and let it sit covered for 5 minutes.
- While the rice is cooking, heat the olive oil in a large skillet over medium heat. Add the diced red onion and garlic, and sauté for 2-3 minutes until softened.
- Stir in the cumin and chili powder, cooking for an additional minute until fragrant.
- Add the black beans, corn, and diced red bell pepper to the skillet. Stir to combine and cook for 5-7 minutes, until heated through. Season with salt and pepper to taste.
- Fluff the cooked brown rice with a fork and divide it among four bowls. Top each bowl with the black bean and vegetable mixture, diced avocado, and halved cherry tomatoes.
- Sprinkle with chopped cilantro and serve with lime wedges on the side for squeezing over the top.

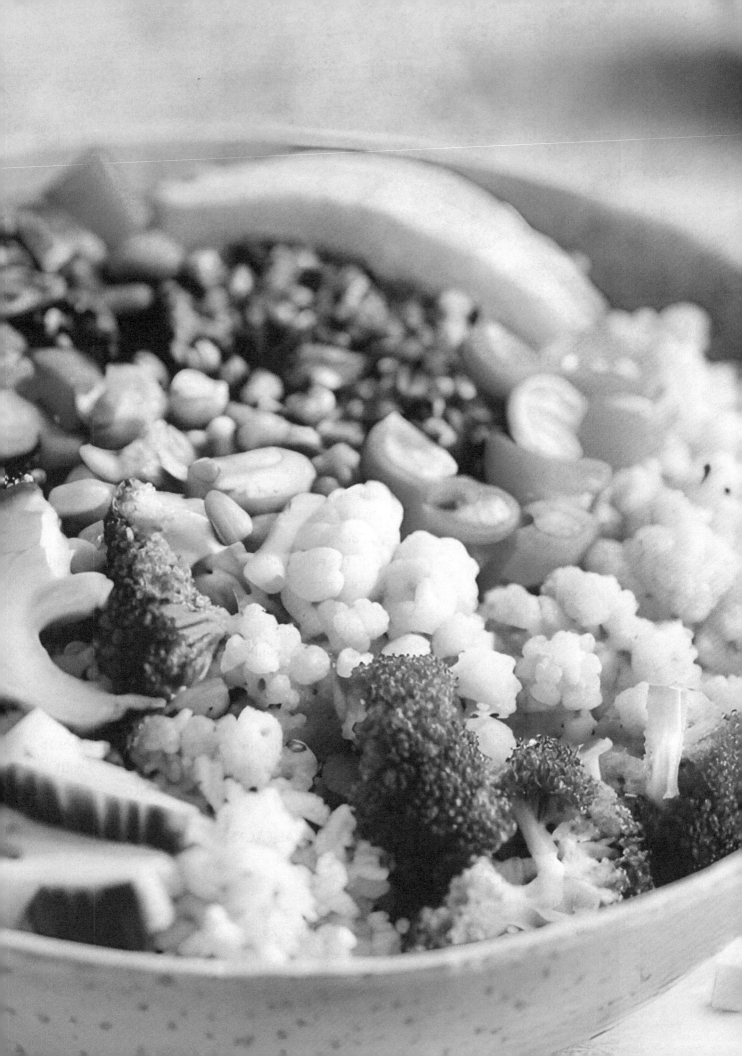

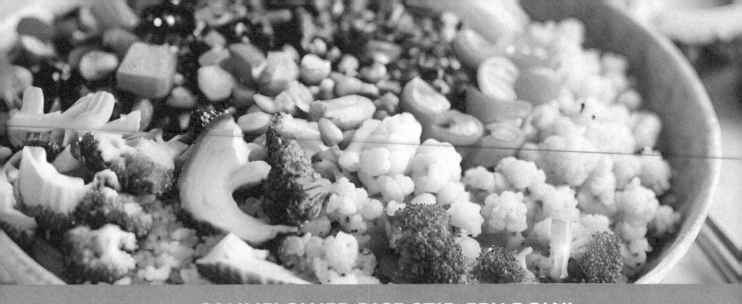

CAULIFLOWER RICE STIR-FRY BOWL

Prep Time: 10 Min | **Cook Time: 15 Min** | **Serving Size: 4**

INGREDIENTS:

- 1 medium head of cauliflower, riced (about 4 cups)
- 1 tablespoon olive oil or avocado oil
- 1 cup bell peppers, diced (red, yellow, or green)
- 1 cup broccoli florets
- 1 cup snap peas or green beans, trimmed
- 1 small carrot, julienned
- 3 green onions, sliced
- 2 cloves garlic, minced
- 1 tablespoon ginger, minced
- 2 tablespoons low-sodium soy sauce or tamari
- 1 tablespoon sesame oil
- 1 tablespoon rice vinegar
- Salt and pepper to taste
- Optional toppings: sesame seeds, chopped cilantro, or crushed red pepper flakes

INSTRUCTIONS:

- If you haven't purchased pre-riced cauliflower, cut the cauliflower into florets and pulse in a food processor until it resembles rice. Set aside.
- In a large skillet or wok, heat the olive oil over medium-high heat.
- Add the garlic and ginger, stirring for about 30 seconds until fragrant. Add the bell peppers, broccoli, snap peas (or green beans), and carrot. Sauté for about 5-7 minutes until the vegetables are tender-crisp.
- Stir in the riced cauliflower, soy sauce, sesame oil, and rice vinegar. Cook for another 5-7 minutes, stirring frequently, until the cauliflower is tender but not mushy.
- Add green onions, and season with salt and pepper to taste. Remove from heat. Serve warm, topped with optional sesame seeds, cilantro, or red pepper flakes.

NUTRITIONAL FACTS

- Calories: 150kcal
- Protein: 5g
- Fat: 7g
- Carbohydrates: 20g
- Fiber: 6g
- Sugars: 3g

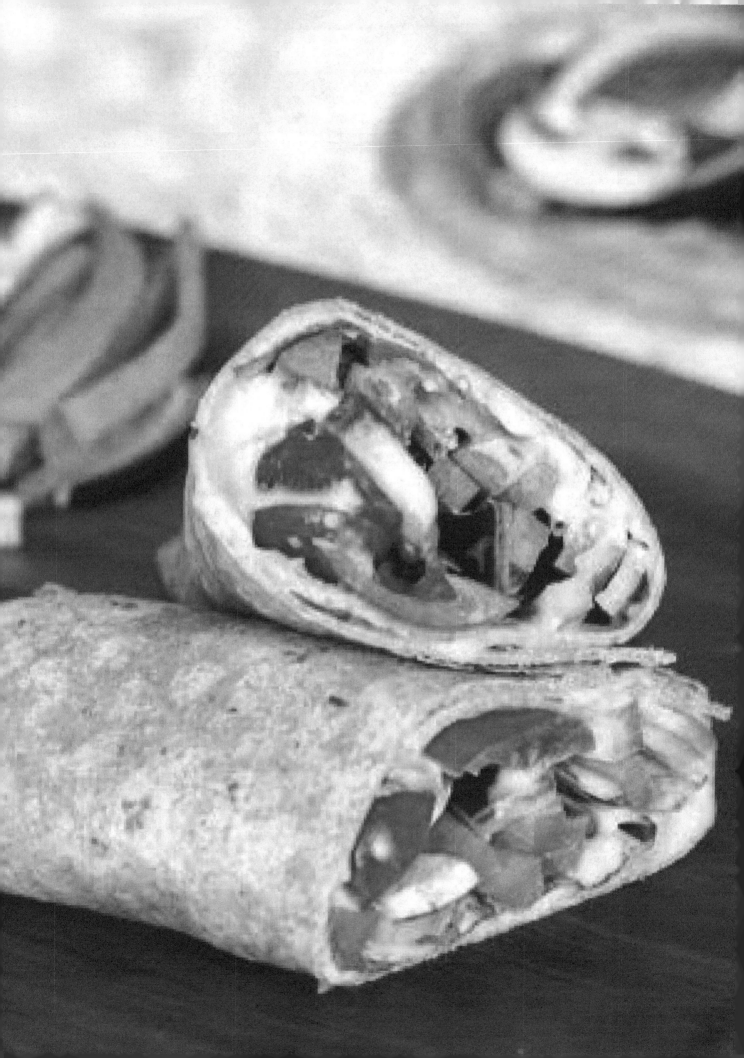

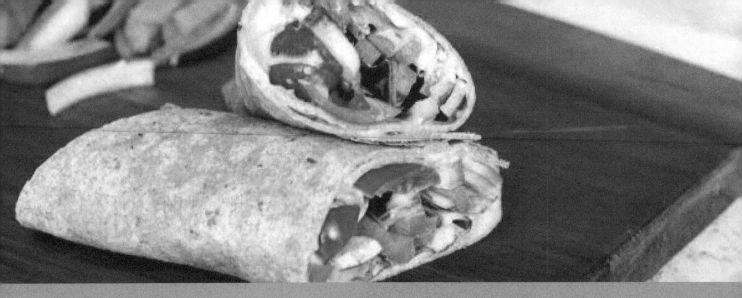

HUMMUS AND VEGGIE WRAP

Prep Time: 10 Min | **Cook Time: 0 Min** | **Serving Size: 1**

INGREDIENTS:

- 1 large whole grain or gluten-free wrap
- 1/2 cup hummus (store-bought or homemade)
- 1/4 cup shredded carrots
- 1/4 cup cucumber, thinly sliced
- 1/4 cup bell pepper, thinly sliced (any color)
- 1/4 cup spinach or mixed greens
- 2 tablespoons avocado, sliced
- 1 tablespoon lemon juice
- Salt and pepper, to taste
- Optional: fresh herbs (e.g., parsley, cilantro), sprouts, or feta cheese for added flavor

NUTRITIONAL FACTS

- Calories: 320
- Total Fat: 12g
- Total Carbohydrates: 45g
- Dietary Fiber: 10g
- Sugars: 5g
- Protein: 10g

INSTRUCTIONS:

- Lay the whole grain or gluten-free wrap flat on a clean surface or plate.
- Evenly spread the hummus over the entire surface of the wrap, leaving about half an inch around the edges.
- Layer the shredded carrots, cucumber slices, bell pepper slices, spinach or mixed greens, and avocado on one half of the wrap.
- Drizzle lemon juice over the vegetables and season with salt and pepper to taste. Add any optional toppings, such as fresh herbs or feta cheese.
- Starting from the side with the veggies, carefully roll the wrap tightly. Make sure to tuck in the sides as you roll to keep the filling from spilling out.
- Slice the wrap in half diagonally. Serve immediately or wrap in foil or parchment paper for an on-the-go option.

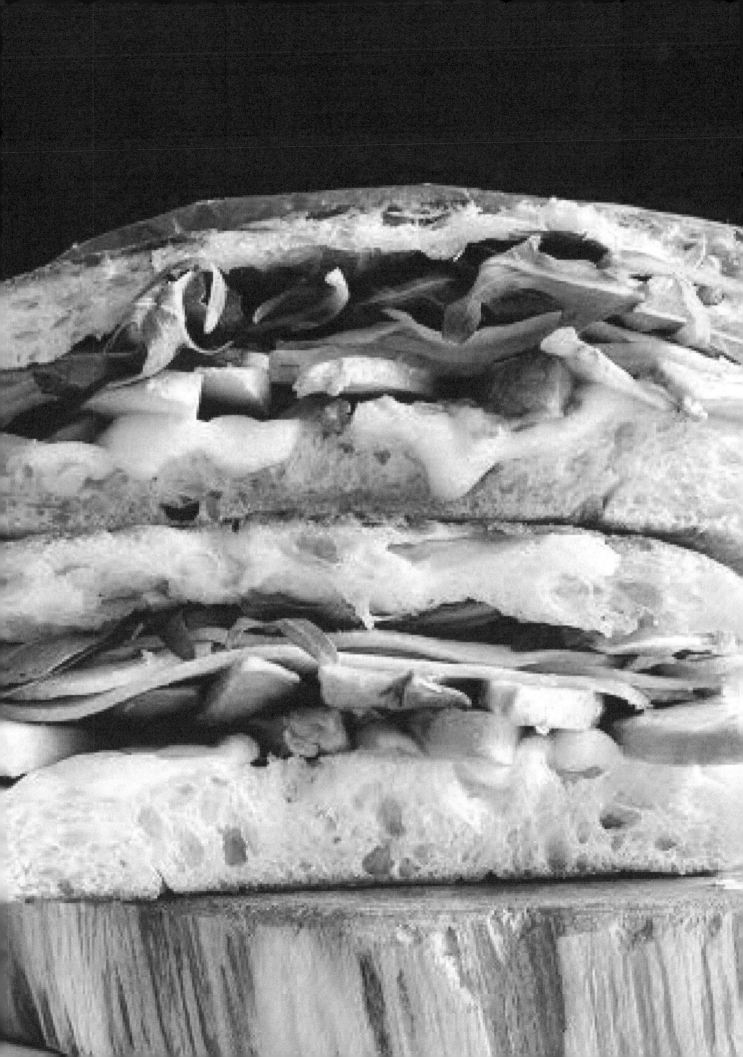

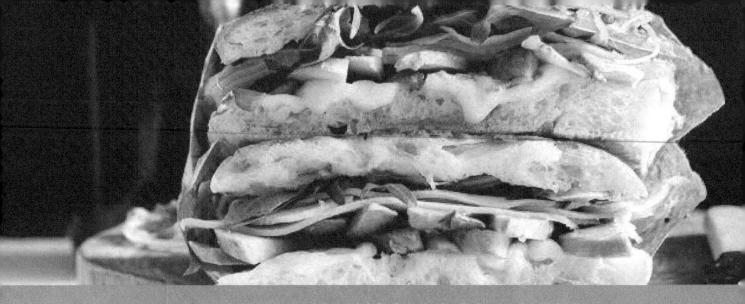

TURKEY AND AVOCADO SANDWICH

Prep Time: 10 Min	Cook Time: 0 Min	Serving Size: 1

INGREDIENTS:

- 2 slices of whole grain or sprouted grain bread
- 4 ounces of sliced turkey breast (preferably organic or nitrate-free)
- 1/2 medium avocado, sliced
- 1 cup fresh spinach or arugula
- 1/4 cup sliced tomatoes
- 1 tablespoon mustard (optional)
- 1 tablespoon hummus (optional)
- Salt and pepper to taste

NUTRITIONAL FACTS

- Calories: 350
- Protein: 26g
- Carbohydrates: 30g
- Dietary Fiber: 10g
- Sugars: 2g
- Fat: 14g

INSTRUCTIONS:

- Wash the spinach or arugula and slice the avocado and tomatoes.
- If using, spread mustard or hummus on one or both slices of bread for added flavor and health benefits.
- On one slice of bread, layer the sliced turkey breast evenly.
- Add the spinach or arugula on top of the turkey.
- Place the sliced avocado on the greens, followed by the sliced tomatoes.
- Sprinkle salt and pepper to taste.
- Place the second slice of bread on top, press gently, and cut the sandwich in half if desired.
- Enjoy your turkey and avocado sandwich as a nutritious meal or snack!

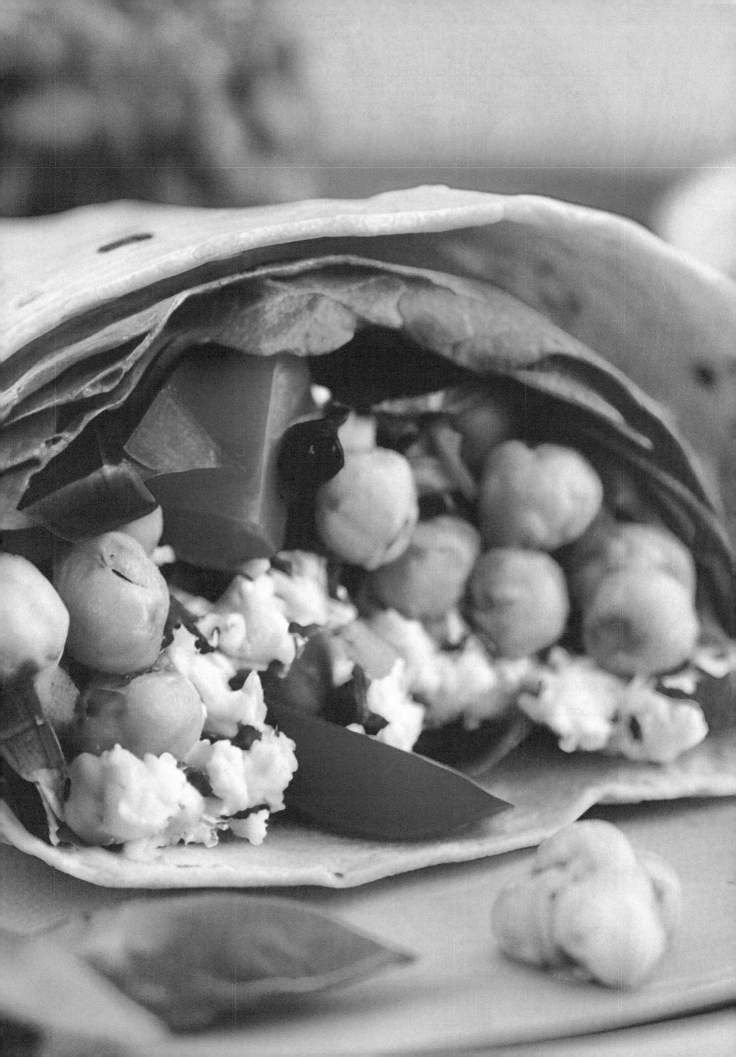

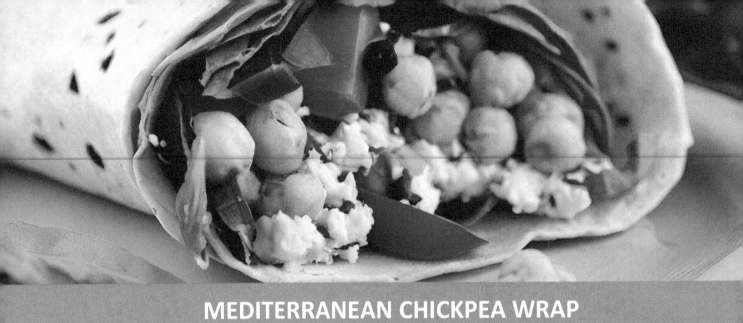

MEDITERRANEAN CHICKPEA WRAP

Prep Time: 15 Min | **Cook Time: 0 Min** | **Serving Size: 2 Wraps**

INGREDIENTS:

- 1 can (15 oz) chickpeas, drained and rinsed
- 1 small cucumber, diced
- 1 small tomato, diced
- 1/4 red onion, thinly sliced
- 1/4 cup Kalamata olives, pitted and chopped
- 1/4 cup crumbled feta cheese (optional)
- 2 tablespoons extra-virgin olive oil
- 1 tablespoon lemon juice
- 1 teaspoon dried oregano
- 2 large whole-wheat wraps
- 1/2 cup fresh spinach or mixed greens
- Salt and pepper, to taste

INSTRUCTIONS:

- In a large bowl, mash half of the chickpeas with a fork or potato masher, leaving some whole for texture.
- Add cucumber, tomato, red onion, olives, and feta cheese (if using) to the bowl with the chickpeas.
- In a small bowl, whisk together the olive oil, lemon juice, oregano, salt, and pepper. Pour the dressing over the chickpea mixture and toss to combine.
- Lay the whole-wheat wraps flat and divide the spinach or mixed greens evenly between them.
- Spoon the chickpea mixture over the greens, then fold the sides of the wrap and roll it up tightly.
- Serve immediately, or wrap in foil for an easy, on-the-go meal.

NUTRITIONAL FACTS

- Calories: 345
- Total Fat: 16g
- Total Carbohydrates: 42g
- Dietary Fiber: 10g
- Sugars: 4g
- Protein: 10g

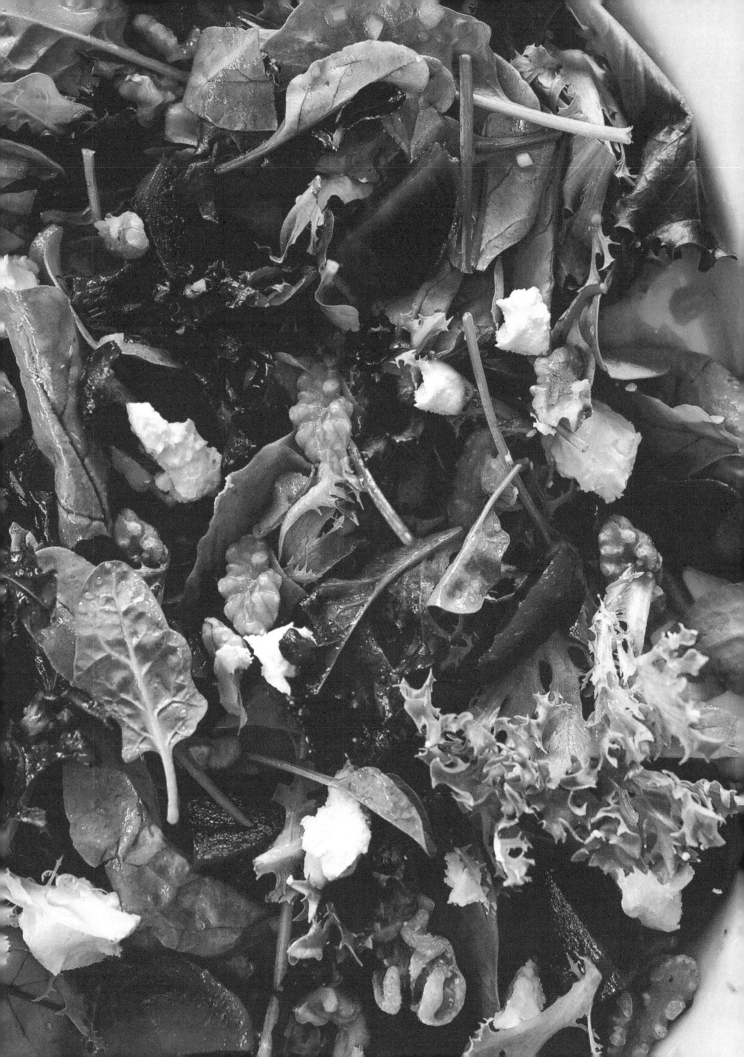

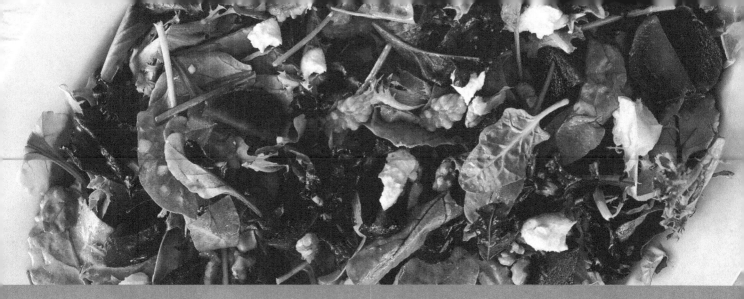

ROASTED BEET AND GOAT CHEESE SALAD

Prep Time: 15 Min | **Cook Time: 45 Min** | **Serving Size: 4**

INGREDIENTS:

- 4 medium beets, trimmed and scrubbed
- 4 cups mixed greens (arugula, spinach, or baby kale)
- 1/4 cup crumbled goat cheese
- 1/4 cup chopped walnuts (optional)
- 1 tablespoon extra virgin olive oil
- 1 tablespoon balsamic vinegar
- 1 teaspoon Dijon mustard
- Salt and pepper to taste
- Fresh herbs for garnish (optional: parsley or chives)

NUTRITIONAL FACTS

- Calories: 180kcal
- Protein: 6g
- Carbohydrates: 14g
- Sugars: 9g
- Fat: 12g
- Fiber: 4g

INSTRUCTIONS:

- Preheat your oven to 400°F (200°C).
- Wrap each beet individually in aluminum foil and place them on a baking sheet.
- Roast the beets for 40-45 minutes, or until they are tender when pierced with a fork.
- Allow the beets to cool, then peel and slice them into wedges or cubes.
- In a small bowl, whisk together the olive oil, balsamic vinegar, Dijon mustard, salt, and pepper until emulsified.
- Arrange the mixed greens on a large serving plate or in individual bowls.
- Top the greens with the roasted beet slices, crumbled goat cheese, and chopped walnuts.
- Drizzle the dressing over the salad, and toss lightly to coat.
- Garnish with fresh herbs if desired.
- Serve immediately.

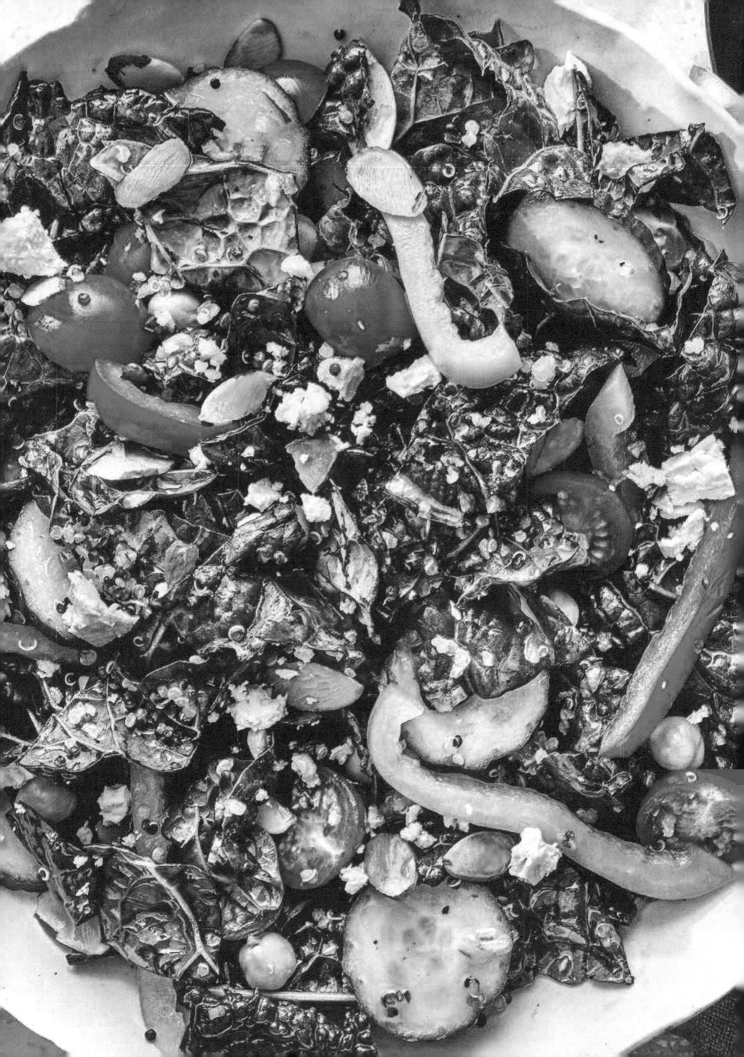

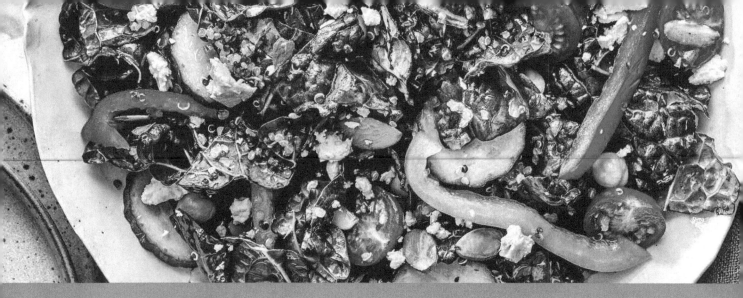

QUINOA AND KALE SALAD WITH LEMON TAHINI DRESSING

Prep Time: 15 Min | **Cook Time: 15 Min** | **Serving Size: 4**

INGREDIENTS:

- For the Salad:
- 1 cup quinoa (uncooked)
- 2 cups water
- 4 cups kale, chopped and de-stemmed
- 1 cucumber, diced
- 1/2 red onion, thinly sliced
- 1/2 cup cherry tomatoes, halved
- 1/4 cup sunflower seeds
- 1 avocado, sliced
- For the Lemon Tahini Dressing:
- 1/4 cup tahini
- 2 tbsp fresh lemon juice
- 1 tbsp apple cider vinegar
- 1 tbsp olive oil
- 1 garlic clove, minced
- 2 tbsp water (to thin the dressing)
- Salt and pepper to taste

INSTRUCTIONS:

- Rinse the quinoa under cold water. Combine quinoa and water in a medium pot and bring to a boil.
- Reduce heat, cover, and simmer for 12-15 minutes until water is absorbed and quinoa is fluffy.
- Let it cool slightly.
- While quinoa is cooking, massage the chopped kale with a small pinch of salt for 2-3 minutes to soften it. Set aside.
- In a small bowl, whisk together tahini, lemon juice, apple cider vinegar, olive oil, minced garlic, and water until smooth.
- Add salt and pepper to taste. Adjust the thickness of the dressing by adding more water if needed.
- In a large bowl, combine the cooked quinoa, massaged kale, cucumber, red onion, and cherry tomatoes.
- Drizzle the lemon tahini dressing over the salad and toss to combine.
- Top with sunflower seeds and sliced avocado just before serving.

NUTRITIONAL FACTS

- Calories: 310 kcal | Carbs: 34g
- Protein: 8g | Fat: 18g
- Fiber: 7g | Sugar: 3g

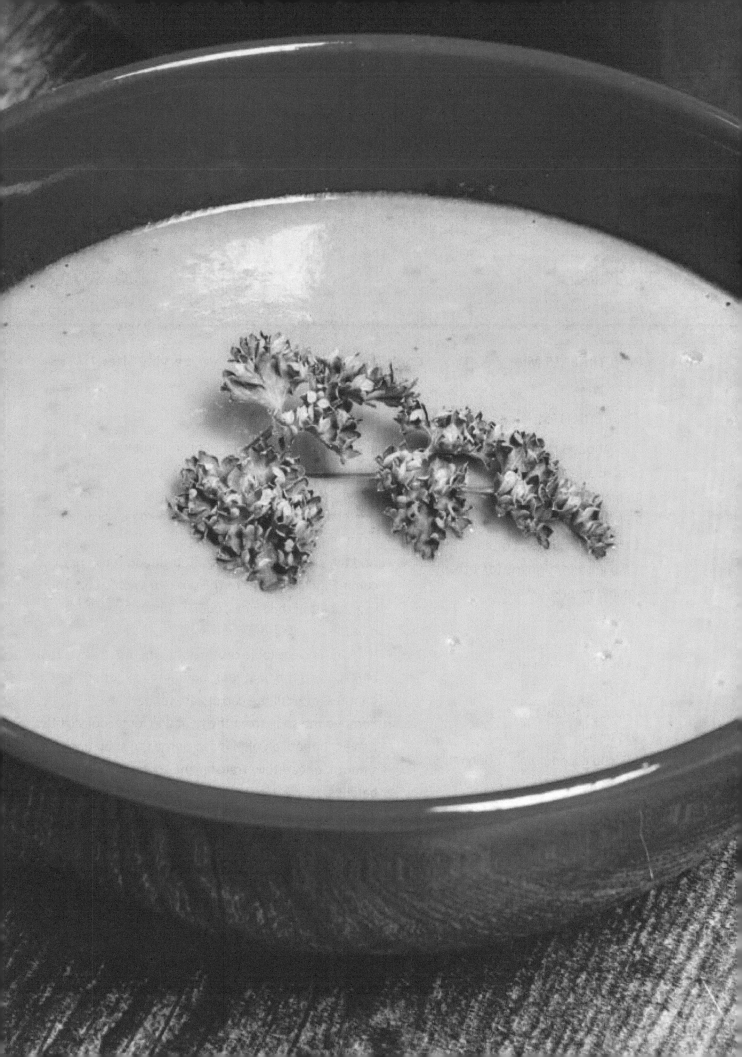

CONCLUSION

Achieving and maintaining optimal cellular health is a long-term, holistic journey that goes beyond individual meals. It's about making conscious, informed decisions every day to support your body's trillions of cells and their intricate functions. A cellular health lifestyle is rooted in consistency—building habits that enhance energy production, repair damage, reduce inflammation, and detoxify the body. The food you eat is the foundation, but there are other key factors that complement nutrition in promoting cellular longevity.

- **Balanced Nutrition**

Nutrient-dense foods, rich in vitamins, minerals, and antioxidants, form the cornerstone of cellular health. Consuming a variety of colorful fruits and vegetables ensures a broad spectrum of phytochemicals, while including healthy fats, lean proteins, and fiber enhances cellular repair, hormone regulation, and gut health. Prioritize whole, unprocessed foods while minimizing refined sugars, unhealthy fats, and artificial additives that can damage cells and accelerate aging.

- **Hydration**

Water is essential for every cellular function, from energy production to waste removal. Proper hydration ensures that nutrients can enter cells efficiently and that toxins can be flushed out. Dehydration impairs cellular metabolism and can lead to a buildup of waste products, increasing oxidative stress. Incorporating hydrating foods like cucumbers, watermelon, and celery, along with drinking water throughout the day, is vital for maintaining healthy cells.

- **Physical Activity**

Regular exercise promotes cellular health in numerous ways. It increases blood flow, delivering more oxygen and nutrients to cells, while stimulating autophagy, the process by which cells clean out damaged components and regenerate. Exercise also boosts the production of mitochondria, the energy factories of cells, making them more efficient in producing ATP (adenosine triphosphate). Engaging in activities like aerobic exercise, strength training, and flexibility exercises supports cellular vitality and overall longevity.

- **Sleep and Cellular Repair**

Sleep is a critical time for cellular repair and regeneration. During deep sleep stages, the body increases the production of growth hormones that stimulate tissue repair, immune function, and the removal of toxins that accumulate in the brain. Poor sleep is linked to increased oxidative stress, inflammation, and impaired cellular function. Prioritizing quality sleep (7-9 hours per night) helps ensure that your cells can perform optimally.

- **Stress Management**

Chronic stress elevates cortisol levels, which can impair immune function and lead to increased cellular damage through inflammation and oxidative stress. Stress management techniques like mindfulness, meditation, yoga, and deep breathing exercises help reduce cortisol levels, allowing cells to function in a more balanced, low-stress environment. Incorporating regular stress-reducing practices into your lifestyle is key to protecting your cells and promoting longevity.

- **Toxin Reduction**

Everyday exposure to environmental toxins—such as pollutants, pesticides, and chemicals in household products—can cause cellular damage. These toxins increase oxidative stress and inflammation, leading to long-term health issues. Adopting a toxin-reducing lifestyle includes choosing organic, chemical-free products, reducing plastic use, and consuming foods that support detoxification, such as cruciferous vegetables, cilantro, and green tea.

By integrating these habits into your daily routine, you can build a lifestyle that fosters cellular health from the inside out. It's not just about living longer, but about living better—with more energy, vitality, and resilience against disease.

MAINTAINING LONGEVITY THROUGH NUTRITION AND DAILY HABITS

Longevity is about more than simply extending your lifespan; it's about extending your health span—the period of life spent in good health, free from chronic disease and frailty. Central to this is the maintenance of cellular health, which, as we've explored, can be significantly influenced by your nutrition and daily habits. Here are some strategies to help you sustain cellular health and longevity over time:

1. Eat for the Long Haul
2. Cycle Through Nutrient-Rich Phases
3. Stay Active Throughout Your Life
4. Focus on Gut Health
5. Mind-Body Connection
6. Monitor and Adapt

GLOSSARY OF NUTRITIONAL TERMS

- **Antioxidants**: Compounds that neutralize free radicals in the body, reducing oxidative stress and protecting cells from damage. Examples include vitamin C, vitamin E, and flavonoids.
- **Autophagy**: A cellular process where cells clean out damaged components and regenerate by breaking down unnecessary or dysfunctional proteins and organelles.
- **Free Radicals:** Unstable molecules that can damage cells and contribute to aging and diseases. These are often produced as a byproduct of metabolism or exposure to environmental toxins.
- **Inflammation**: A natural response by the immune system to injury or infection. Chronic inflammation, however, can damage cells and tissues, leading to a variety of diseases.
- **Mitochondria**: Organelles within cells that generate energy in the form of ATP. Healthy mitochondria are crucial for cellular energy production and overall vitality.
- **Omega-3 Fatty Acids:** Essential fats that the body cannot produce on its own. They are anti-inflammatory and are important for heart, brain, and cellular membrane health.
- **Phytochemicals**: Compounds found in plants that have protective or disease-preventing properties. Examples include flavonoids, carotenoids, and polyphenols.
- **Telomeres**: Protective caps at the ends of chromosomes that prevent DNA from fraying during cell division. Shortened telomeres are associated with aging and an increased risk of disease.
- **Oxidative Stress:** An imbalance between free radicals and antioxidants in the body, which can lead to cell and tissue damage.

MEASUREMENT CONVERSIONS

In many recipes, accurate measurements are essential for ensuring the right balance of ingredients. Here are some common measurement conversions to help you navigate the recipes in this cookbook:

- **Volume Conversions:**
  - 1 teaspoon (tsp) = 5 milliliters (ml)
  - 1 tablespoon (tbsp) = 15 milliliters (ml)
  - 1 cup = 240 milliliters (ml)
  - 1 pint = 473 milliliters (ml)
  - 1 quart = 946 milliliters (ml)
  - 1 gallon = 3.78 liters (L)

- **Weight Conversions:**
- 1 ounce (oz) = 28.35 grams (g)
- 1 pound (lb) = 454 grams (g)
- 1 kilogram (kg) = 1000 grams (g)

- **Temperature Conversions:**
- Celsius (°C) to Fahrenheit (°F): (°C × 9/5) + 32 = °F
- Fahrenheit (°F) to Celsius (°C): (°F − 32) × 5/9 = °C

By referencing these conversions, you'll be able to prepare meals with precision and consistency, whether you're using metric or imperial systems.

NOTES

Made in the USA
Las Vegas, NV
24 November 2024

12523829R00044